2nd EDITION

Understanding

and

Preventing

AIDS

A
Book
for
Everyone

A Publication of Health Alert Press

Copyright © 1988 by Chris Jennings

Health Alert Press
P.O. Box 2060
Cambridge, MA 02238-2060
(617) 497-4190

ISBN 0-936571-01-2

Library of Congress Catalog Card Number: 87-80364

To my parents,
Zachariah Alexander Jennings and Grace Elaine Jennings

Acknowledgements

Special thanks belong to my sister, Karen Jennings, for assuming all the burden.

Belated thanks to Dr. Robert Schooley, Dr. Joe Sodrowski, Dr. Ken Mayer, and Dr. John Beldekas for their valuable time and contributions which made the first edition of this book possible.

My most sincere gratitude to Priscilla Battis, Phoebe Leed, and Nathan Neel for their time, knowledge, perspective, support, and particularly for appearing, at the most trying times, with a cup of coffee and a bowl of soup.

Table of Contents

List of Figures

Preface

AIDS is a disease that will affect, directly or indirectly, virtually every living person in the world. Beyond being a disease, AIDS is a social force of major historical importance. Worldwide, AIDS will leave its mark on law, education, medicine, science, and social behavior.

While we live in a world of mass communication, mass hysteria still rules, at least regarding AIDS. Despite the abundance of media attention awarded to AIDS, extremely few individuals have a grasp of the essential facts. Moreover, even fewer individuals know how these facts relate to their well-being or degree of personal risk. This lack of understanding stems from the built-in limitations of the media and public health agencies in distributing information about sex and drugs, and from our society's erosion of trust in medical, scientific, and political authority figures.

AIDS has such far-reaching effect that an in-depth understanding of its nature cannot be left to the medical profession alone. Nor do all members of the medical profession desire the responsibility of decision-making AIDS has thrust upon them.

Therefore, this book was designed to provide accurate, non-sensationalistic, easy-to-understand information for both medical professionals and laypeople alike. Beyond providing facts, this book creates a framework which outlines the the biological nature of AIDS, the scientific and social aspects of the AIDS epidemic, and how AIDS relates to them as individuals. Briefly stated, this book provides understanding and perspective. The book is designed to be read as a whole, but it can be read in parts, and the index allows it to be used as a reference work.

This book primarily describes the AIDS epidemic as it appears in the United States (with apologies to our many foreign readers). However, the information contained in this book was gleaned from approximately 2000 medical and scientific articles stemming from research performed in the United States, Great Britain, France, Sweden, Germany, and additional European, African and South American countries.

This book is intended for educational use only. Any suggestions or information provided in this book should not be construed as medical advice.

1. Disease, Culture, and Behavior

Due to the public's understanding of AIDS, a person is hard-pressed to discuss AIDS without also mentioning sex or homosexuality in the conversation. More so than any other disease in modern history, AIDS challenges our conceptions of freedom and lifestyle. AIDS is very much a social disease; thus discussions of sex and society are necessary to achieve an understanding of AIDS.

History of Sexually Transmitted Diseases (STDs)

The AIDS epidemic is not the world's first STD epidemic, nor is it the first to drastically change sexual attitudes and behavior. Social attitudes about STDs and sexual behavior have changed throughout history. In general, as observed in the western world, there is a pendulum effect; very strict social codes of sexual behavior and punitive attitudes toward STD patients follow an era of STD epidemics. In time, as the memory and effects of the STD epidemics fade, less strict social and sexual behavior again come into being. The cycle then repeats.

Some historians believe that the puritanical attitudes of the Victorian era (1800s), known for its fear of and secrecy about sex, were the result of widespread syphilis epidemics in the preceding century. These epidemics also changed fashion. White, ponytailed wigs covered heads balding from second-stage syphilis. High, ruffled collars and cuffs covered the spotting of syphilitic wounds.

On the rebound from the Victorian era, most of the western world spent the first half of this century relaxing their sexual views. Then, in the 1950s the current round of STD epidemics began. The United States had its own, almost unnoticed, gonorrhea epidemic, which began in 1957 and continued until 1979. During that period, the number of gonorrhea cases multiplied five times, from 230,000 reported cases in 1957 to over 1 million reported cases in 1979. These were not all the cases, just those reported by doctors. Immediately following the gonorrhea epidemic came the surging rise of herpes and several other STDs which have not received as much media attention.

The supposed "sexual revolution" of the 1960s contributed to the gonorrhea epidemic, but only to a limited degree. Although public attitudes about sex relaxed during the sixties, premarital sex has been increasing steadily in the United States since 1900. The sixties merely continued the trend. The main difference of the sixties was that, perhaps due to new birth control technology, more single women were engaging in premarital sex. The number of men engaging in premarital sex has remained basically the same since the 1940s.

The real causes of the American gonorrhea epidemic occurred in the early 1950s. First, penicillin and other "miracle drugs" were developed, encouraging both the public and the medical profession to lose fear of infectious diseases, including STDs. Since STDs were supposedly curable with a shot or pill, many doctors no longer put substantial effort into tracing their patients' past sexual partners. Wishing to protect their patients' privacy, some doctors also stopped reporting STD cases to the government's recording centers. And, thinking that the STD problem was conquered, the government stopped spending money on anti-STD campaigns (campaigns which peaked during the wars) and instead focused on other public health problems.

Despite the "sexual revolution," the 1960s media maintained a blackout on STDs. For example, the words *gonorrhea* and *syphilis* were removed from ads put out by the American Medical Association to warn people of the dangers of STDs. The ignorance that resulted from this media blackout and from the lack of public education was the major cause of the gonorrhea epidemic.

The occurrence of STDs reveals the differences between ideals, morals, and actual behavior. No single medical treatment or any single social change will eliminate STDs. Controlling STDs requires a realistic understanding of sexual behavior as a normal human impulse. On the part of many individuals, efforts to control the current spread of the AIDS epidemic will challenge their willingness to frankly discuss topics formerly not considered proper for public discussion. Any educational efforts concerning AIDS must address sexual behavior, reproduction, and social values in a manner never before practiced in our society.

The Coming of AIDS

AIDS stands for "*a*cquired *i*mmune *d*eficiency *s*yndrome." AIDS, the leading killer of men aged 20 to 50 in New York City and San Francisco, is the number one health priority of the U.S. Public Health Service.

A "syndrome" is a group of clinical symptoms that make up a disease or abnormal condition. "Clinical" means seen in the doctor's office, not discovered by laboratory tests. In a syndrome not all symptoms have to appear in any one patient. Syndromes may be caused by many things, but in AIDS the syndrome is caused by a defect in the body's immune system. The immune system defends the body against disease.

The diseases of the AIDS syndrome are caused by germs we encounter every day. In fact, some of those germs live permanently, in small numbers, inside the human body. Should the immune (defense) system weaken, these germs have the opportunity to multiply freely, and so the diseases these germs cause are called "opportunistic diseases."

The problem of AIDS, as we understand it now, began in 1981, when five homosexual men in Los Angeles were discovered to have *Pneumocystis carinii* pneumonia (PCP). PCP is usually cured with antibiotic drugs; the PCP in these men, however, resisted drug therapy. PCP also sometimes occurs in kidney transplant patients whose immune systems have been chemically suppressed.

As more cases of mysterious immune-deficiency diseases came into being among more and more homosexual men, doctors guessed that it was an acquired disease, a disease that could be passed from one person to another. The mysterious disease, AIDS, was given its name before its cause was discovered.

Doctors and scientists were baffled. Theories regarding the cause of AIDS have changed over time. At first, scientists thought that some factor in the homosexual lifestyle caused AIDS. Eventually, this line of thought led to the "immune-overload theory." In this theory, the immune system was thought to have collapsed from overwork, that is, from being exposed to too many diseases. The first people to come down with AIDS practiced a number of habits known to increase the likelihood of catching diseases. These habits included having sexual contact with large numbers of people, using large quantities of both legal and illegal drugs, and having irregular sleeping and eating habits.

The immune-overload theory was eventually rejected as scientists found evidence that AIDS was caused by an infectious agent (germ) that could be passed from one person to another. First, doctors found that sexual partners of AIDS patients were coming down with AIDS. Then it was discovered that intravenous (IV) drug users, who use syringes to inject drugs into their bodies (shoot up), were also coming down with AIDS.

Finally, in May 1983, Dr. Luc Montagnier of the Pasteur Institute in Paris obtained a virus from an AIDS patient which he believed to cause AIDS. He named it the "Lymphadenopathy-Associated Virus," or LAV for short, because it was isolated from a lymph node (gland). Lymphadenopathy is a condition related to AIDS. Few other scientists believed Dr. Montagnier, though, and lacking the resources to continue studying the virus, he placed his samples on ice. Then, in May 1984, Dr. Robert Gallo of the National Cancer Institute in Bethesda, Maryland, also isolated an AIDS-related virus, the "Human T-cell Lymphotropic Virus," or HTLV-III. *Lymphotropic* means that the virus likes to grow in lymphocytes, a certain type of white blood cell. The LAV/HTLV-III virus was also named the "AIDS-Related Virus," or ARV, by Dr. Joe Levy of the University of California.

The variety of names caused confusion and dispute. By scientific tradition, the discoverers of a new organism get to name it (often after themselves). However, there is an ongoing legal dispute between the Pasteur Institute and the National Cancer Institute over who first isolated and identified the virus. Besides the right to name the virus, millions of dollars are at stake. The discoverer of the virus (or his institute) will receive royalties from all sales of AIDS-testing kits worldwide.

In 1986, the International Committee on the Taxonomy of Viruses attempted to simplify things by giving the LAV/HTLV-III/ARV virus yet another name. "Taxonomy" is the science of naming living things. The committee's new name for the virus is the "Human Immunodeficiency Virus," or HIV for short. The acronym HIV is used throughout this book because it has been adopted by the media and by the U.S. Public Health Service in most of its publications.

The Uses of Sex

Sex is nature's way of creating *diversity* in organisms that use sex to make offspring. The wonder of sexual reproduction is that each individual offspring is unique, differing from every other individual. For example, humans at birth are capable of expressing all possible behaviors existing in the human universe, each in his or her own way. The human's environment will determine the individual's language and greatly affect the individual's options and viewpoint of the world. Genetic diversity is advantageous. With diversity, it becomes less likely that one disease will wipe out all humans and more likely that one person in a group will have the answer.

Figure 1: Who's Who in STDs

Historical figures who allegedly contracted sexually transmitted diseases.

Kings, Emperors & Politicians

Friedrich der Grosse a.k.a. Frederick the Great 1712–1786	King of Prussia, his military campaigns and diplomatic ploys made Prussia the greatest military force of Europe. He liberalized religion, lessened the use of censorship and torture, and promoted French language and culture among nobles.
Ivan Vasilyevich Grozny a.k.a. Ivan the Terrible 1530–1584	Russian czar known for his reign of terror. Sought to bring Russia into the European theater of nations.
Francois D'Angouleme a.k.a. Francis I 1494–1547	French King, the first of five monarchs of his line. A humanist and patron of the Renaissance arts and scholarship, he fought a series of wars with the Holy Roman Empire.
Charles Le Bien-Servi a.k.a. Charles the Well-Served, or The Victorious 1403–1461	The French King who succeeded in driving the English from French soil with the help of Joan of Arc.
Napoleon Bonaparte a.k.a. Napoleon, Napoleon I, The Little Corporal 1769–1821	The Corsican-born general who eventually became Emperor of the French Empire. A brilliant military strategist, he revolutionized military organization, education, and government.
Henry VII a.k.a. Henry Tudor, Earl of Richmond 1457–1485	The English King who ended the War of the Roses, he founded the Tudor Dynasty.
Edward Albert Christian George Andrew Patrick David a.k.a. Prince Edward, Edward VIII, Duke of Windsor 1894–1972	The Prince of Wales and King of England who abdicated the British throne to marry an American commoner.
Woodrow Wilson 1856–1924	The 28th President of the United States, serving two terms. An idealist, he first tried to maintain U.S. neutrality and then led the U.S. into World War I. He was a major promoter of the League of Nations.
Vladimir Lenin a.k.a. Lenin 1870–1924	Founder of the Russian Communist Party, a leader of the Bolshevik Revolution, first head of the modern Soviet government, noted political writer and philosopher. He created the official Communist ideology of the Soviet Union based on the ideas of philosopher Karl Marx.

Artists, Composers & Philosophers

Robert Schumann 1810–1856	German composer renowned for his piano music, songs, and orchestral arrangements.
Ludwig van Beethoven a.k.a. Beethoven 1770–1827	German composer, a student of Wolfgang Amadeus Mozart. His works stand as some of the greatest in classical music.
Paul Gauguin 1848–1903	One of leading French painters of the Post-impressionist period, famous for his depictions of Tahiti.
Fyodor Mikhaylovich Dostoyevsky a.k.a. Dostoyevsky 1821–1881	Russian writer of novels and short stories. He was imprisoned in Siberia for participating in radical discussion groups. His most famous novels are *Crime and Punishment* and *Brothers Karamazov*.
Francisco de Goya a.k.a. Goya 1746–1828	Spanish artist who influenced 19th and 20th century painters. His paintings recorded the upheavals of his time, including the Napoleonic invasion.
Willem van Gogh a.k.a. Van Gogh 1853–1890	The Dutch painter who greatly influenced Expressionism. His most famous work is *The Starry Night*. Physical and mental illness eventually led to his suicide.
Johann Wolfgang von Goethe a.k.a. Goethe 1749–1832	German novelist, playwright, poet, and philosopher whose works are studied in universities around the world today.

Popes and Cardinals

Cardinal Armand-Jean De Richelieu a.k.a. The Red Eminence 1585–1542	A ruthless, powerful, religious and political figure who suppressed certain religious elements out of political necessity; outlawed dueling among French nobles; and eventually found himself in opposition to the Pope for political reasons.
Cardinal Thomas Wolsey 1475–1530	A lowborn cardinal and statesmen of England who became influential in the court of Henry VIII. Together they planned to make England the major power of Europe. Court intrigue contributed to his downfall.
Giovanni Maria Ciocchi Del Monte a.k.a. Pope Julius III 1487–1555	Pope from 1550 to 1555, he saw the need for reform in the Church, tried to keep the cardinals within monastic life, and was a patron of Renaissance thought. Built the Church of St. Andrew in Rome with Michelangelo as architect.
Alessandro Ottaviano De' Medici a.k.a. Pope Leo XI 1535–1605	Pope for a month, from April 1, 1605 to April 27.

As a species (a group of organisms that breed with each other) humans are very successful. All living organisms try to live and reproduce. These functions are genetically programmed into all living creatures. The reproductive drive is affected by environmental conditions, such as food supply and shelter, for the organisms that need it. In humans, the "environment" includes one's culture. Humans are probably unique in that, more and more, our survival depends on social programming (culture), not genetic programming.

Humans breed so successfully that not every instance of sexual intercourse needs to be an attempt at making babies. Nor do all living humans need to reproduce. Humans are spread across all parts and climates of the earth, with greater numbers of new humans arriving every year. Thus in human societies, sex has gained symbolic purposes not directly connected with reproduction. These alternative purposes of sexual activity are strongly woven into the human social fiber. Besides using it to make babies, people use sex for fun, for money, as an expression of love, as the foundation for a bond, as an expression of power, for ego fulfillment, and for stress release, to name a few. From a biological viewpoint, sexual actions performed for these purposes are mock sex. "Mock" is used in the biological sense here, loosely defined as "not used for its primary biological function."

In most organisms, reproduction is limited by food supply or inability to find a mate. Humans are such successful survivors that there have been few biological restraints on human reproduction. Rather, cultural mating rituals and taboos are instituted to control sexual activity. Taboos are rules which forbid certain activities, not necessarily sexual, and are often related to eating habits. In humans, social conditioning overcomes basic genetic engineering. A Hindu might starve to death rather than eat a sacred cow; a Christian might refrain from sex rather than go to hell.

Historically, taboos often stem either from history's biological lessons or social needs. For example, a biological lesson learned very early by humans was not to urinate or defecate near the water supply. Another lesson learned early was that mating between brother and sister was likely to produce sickly, deformed, and mentally retarded children. Mating between first cousins is also risky, but some marginal societies, which have few individuals of breeding age, allow marriage between first cousins.

Taboos often last longer than people's memory of why the taboo exists. Sometimes the original reason a taboo exists is forgotten and people have to make up a new reason to support it. Some taboos outlive their usefulness. Other taboos may be eternal. Some taboos have to be constantly relearned, particularly, it seems, the ones about keeping wastes away from water.

Homosexuals. For the purpose of this book, a "homosexual" is a person who has engaged in any sexual activity with a person of the same sex. The number of sexual encounters, one or one thousand, does not matter. Homosexuality is not necessarily a permanent trait. Many adolescent individuals, particularly males, at some point in adolescence engage in homosexual experimentation or experience adoration, bordering on obsession, for individuals of the same sex.

Homosexuality and homosexual acts have probably been around since humans have existed. For some long forgotten reason, homosexuality and homosexual behavior is a strong taboo in many cultures—not all.

The number of homosexuals in a society may never vary. However, the number of "practicing" homosexuals in a society probably depends on many factors, culture and economy probably being the most important. In terms of culture, tolerance of individual differences is the important variable. Even in the United States, a number of regional cultures exist, varying in their tolerance of homosexuality or any other behavior off the norm. In many regions, the gun, the bomb, and the torch are still commonly used to establish community standards.

From the economic point of view, agricultural societies might be less likely to tolerate homosexuality, since the production of offspring, to work the farms and support parents in their old age, is a priority.

In the United States, the open expression of homosexuality seems related to population density. In general, only in large cities do many homosexuals feel comfortable being identified publicly as homosexual. Presumably, this open expression is related to the tolerance of city dwellers for different lifestyles, perhaps stemming from the anonymity of living in a city away from restraining family and community ties, pressures, and roles.

There are many roads to "homosexuality." Individual people engage in homosexual behaviors for a number of diverse reasons. Some homosexuals feel compelled to engage in homosexual relations, sexual and otherwise. A strong argument exists for a genetic basis for homosexuality, that, in some people, homosexuality is an inherited trait. Another viewpoint is that, at birth, all humans are capable of expressing all human behaviors, and that the individual human's environment determines the individual's mold.

This is the old "nature versus nurture" controversy. However, a merging of the two opposing concepts is possible. Every individual has a different threshold at which certain behaviors are expressed. One person exposed to a certain set of circumstances may express homosexuality while a second under the same circumstances does not, but may under other circumstances.

It is true that among specific populations of homosexuals, certain recurrent psychological themes exist, such as emotional distance from their biological families and problems with compulsive behavior, including sex, alcohol, and other drug use. Again, this is some—not all—homosexuals. The thing to remember is that all homosexuals are individuals. The term "homosexual" encompasses people who actively engage in sex, people who do not engage in sex, people who devote their lives to sex, and people who devote their lives to sports, people compelled by love or some inner force to bond with same-sex individuals, and people who are "homosexual" purely for the sexual experience or purely for the enjoyment of shocking other people.

In truth, sexual orientation is only a small part of a person's life. A homosexual person does not necessarily function differently from a heterosexual person in any nonsexual social function.

Bisexuals. Some people are "bisexuals," people who engage in sexual activity with both males and females. Again, there are many roads to bisexuality, and bisexuality need not be a permanant state of being. Presumably, many individuals engage in sexual experimentation with same-sex individuals, doing so purely for the sexual experience.

Bisexual males, as a group, may present a problem. Reportedly, many bisexual males are not comfortable with the homosexual portion of their personalities (of course, many are). Many bisexual men are married and have families. A common theme in these situations is that the bisexual male has homosexual "binges," often associated with alcohol (or other drug) use. Alcohol, of course, lowers the inhibitions. Commonly, these men experience extreme guilt and shame after these binges and swear off the experience—until next time.

In one viewpoint, these types of bisexual males are "really" homosexuals, who hide their homosexual behavior from themselves by engaging in group sex with both male(s) and female(s) present and then calling it "just a little kinky sex," rather than acknowledging the homosexual aspect of it. In a similar vein, a drug-binging bisexual commonly blames the homosexual behavior on drug use, rather than acknowledging any innate homosexual desire.

Bisexual males probably provide the HIV with the best bridge from the homosexual population to the heterosexual population. Many bisexual men are very secretive about their bisexuality. This population of individuals is difficult to reach, but these individuals and their sexual partners may represent a hidden component of the AIDS epidemic.

The subgroup of bisexuals highlights the problems of a sexually repressive society. Millions of people engage in secretive sexual behaviors, and all these behaviors remain hidden. Consequently, in times of crisis such as the AIDS epidemic, it is impossible to estimate how many individuals are at high risk. There is no way of directly contacting these individuals and little hope of encouraging them to come forward on their own.

Labels and Behavior. Reportedly, many individuals refuse to recognize that they belong to a "high-risk group," denying that they are "homosexual" even though they have sex with same-sex partners. In short, they deny that the label "homosexual" applies to themselves, and in doing so, deny their own elevated risk for exposure to AIDS.

For this reason, AIDS education advocates are placing new emphasis on "high-risk behaviors" and "high-risk activities" rather than stressing the importance of the "high-risk groups." For the purpose of this book, anyone practicing risky behaviors belongs to a high-risk group.

Compulsive Behaviors

Compulsive behaviors are irrational behaviors that a person feels forced to do, often on a regular basis. People who engage in compulsive behaviors are unhealthy, in social and psychological terms. A compulsive behavior may be a normal social behavior, but performed for the wrong reasons, performed at the wrong time, or performed too many times for the good of the people involved. Compulsive behavior is a matter of degree.

For example, food, sex, smoking, or golf can be the centers of compulsive behavior. Taken in moderation, each can be beneficial or only mildly harmful. But the business executive who cannot overcome his compulsion to cancel business meetings and go golfing will soon have social, financial, and, perhaps, emotional problems. Golf in moderation is a beneficial behavior, offering the executive fresh air and exercise. Golf in excess is harmful. The amount of golf a person can handle depends on the individual's occupation (golf pro?), financial status, marital status, and genetic makeup. It's the same issue with chocolate. In fact, many compulsive behaviors center around food.

Compulsive behaviors are based on the need for reward—immediate reward. Virtually all compulsive behaviors give some immediate reward—a "quick fix." Chocolate is sweet, and its sugar affects the metabolism; tobacco tastes good to the habituated taste of the smoker, and the nicotine grants the smoker a "rush," or nicotine high. Sex offers physical pleasure and a menu of mental and emotional pleasures, depending on the individual's emotional makeup.

In developing a pattern of compulsive behaviors, individuals lose their ability to perceive and be satisfied by medium- and long-term goals and the rewards these goals offer. Rather, compulsive people become absorbed in their rituals of compulsive behavior, sometimes to the exclusion of everything else. Some compulsive people are called "addicts."

Not all compulsive people practice their compulsions to extremes. Some people are "weekend" junkies, alcoholics, and chocoholics, able to perform occupational and social functions and limit their habit so it does not harm their health in the short term.

Some people are compulsive about orgasms. These people do not feel good unless they have two, ten, or fifteen orgasms a day. Some males who are called homosexual are really just "sex addicts" or "orgasm addicts." They obtain their orgasms from other compulsive males because these males are easier to deal with; the issues of pregnancy, intimacy, and trust are not important in this form of compulsive sex.

Compulsive behaviors, as a group, are familiar to mental health professionals. A variety of techniques exist for modifying these behaviors and replacing them with healthier habits.

A critical examination of U.S. society reveals that our culture breeds many compulsive people. Compulsive behaviors are normal behaviors which developed into unhealthy habits. In theory, a society that creates a great number of compulsive people is missing some element of cultural education that promotes the choice of healthy habits. People who engage in compulsive behaviors must learn new behaviors to overcome the triggers of compulsion, thought to be stress, isolation, and boredom.

Societies attempt to shape its members into *roles* that fit the social framework. As society becomes more specialized and complex, humans have greater difficulty playing the roles that society creates, because traditional roles have disappeared for many. It is unlikely that society will become less complex with a return to the roles of the past. Thus, society needs to allow greater diversity and greater expression of alternative lifestyles as people try to grow into the new roles of the twenty-first century.

Drug Use

Many drugs serve as a useful focus for compulsive behaviors. Both legal and illegal drugs offer quick-acting rewards which can be obtained relatively inexpensively. The problem of drugs (as opposed to chocolate or sex) is that illegal ones make people into criminals and force them to deal with criminal elements. In fact, the illegality of drugs attracts some individuals to them—the fascination of the forbidden. Also, compulsive use of most drugs quickly damages people's bodies and their mental, emotional, and social faculties.

Some degree of drug use is considered normal in most societies. Alcohol is the traditional drug in western societies. Since alcohol is so common, it is also the first drug many compulsive people encounter. As a result, alcohol addiction is the greatest drug problem in the United States. In 1984 approximately 90,000 alcohol-related deaths were recorded in the United States while cocaine-related deaths numbered around 1500.

Humans are not the only animals that like to use drugs. Rats and some other animals like alcohol, marijuana, and cocaine. Different drugs satisfy different "quick-fix" needs in various individuals. Heroin quickly removes all physical and emotional pain. Cocaine "picks you up" (and also triggers circuitry in the brain that makes one feel rewarded—rats eat cocaine until they overdose). Alcohol makes you "high," "stoned," or "wasted." Better yet, alcohol provides an excuse to do anything one wants. One can always apologize the next day, blaming disagreeable behavior on drunkenness, and usually get away with it.

Interestingly, a person's emotional state and expectations can strongly affect a drug's effects. For example, in research studies, people smoked tobacco "joints," believing them to be marijuana, and reported being "high." Conversely, other people smoked marijuana without effect. In similar settings, heroin addicts reported "rushes" from injections of warm water.

Although the pharmacological (physical) effects of these drugs are real, including actual physical addiction (alcohol's being among the worst) and poisoning, compulsions are based on reward and the control addicts have over the reward. Control is an important issue. The ability to grant themselves this reward may be one of the few things in life that addicts control. Another important factor of drug use is the camaraderie formed by drug users. The social rituals of drug use are very strong.

The Government

Different segments of the government in the U.S. contribute to the fight against AIDS. (See Figure 2.)

The stated goals of the U.S. Public Health Service are (1) to reduce the transmission of HIV infection by 1987; (2) to reduce the increase in the incidence (appearance) of AIDS by 1990; and (3) to eliminate the transmission of HIV by 2000 A.D., with a decline in the incidence of AIDS thereafter.

Public health officials are faced with a difficult situation. Rather than act on a purely scientific or public health basis, they must attempt to control disease while protecting the society's traditional social values. The dual goals of preventing the spread of diseases and upholding traditional social values are often contradictory.

Church and state are constitutionally separate in the United States, but many public health officials must work within laws based on religious moral standards. For example, some public health officials cannot legally promote the use of birth control devices and thus are unable to tell people to use condoms to reduce the risk of HIV transmission. AIDS service organizations and other private and non-profit organizations are relied upon to handle this facet of public education. However, most existing AIDS service organizations necessarily direct their efforts to the homosexual male population. Thus, not every individual is comfortable contacting these organizations for information.

In another situation, government money was withdrawn from AIDS service organizations because AIDS prevention flyers used "dirty words" to describe body parts and sexual acts. Effective education takes place in a language that the students understand. For the intended population, "dirty words" are commonly used and understood. The use of medical and scientific terms may not effectively communicate the necessary information. This withdrawal of funding slowed the distribution of information to certain populations of high-risk individuals and presumably resulted in additional AIDS cases.

While the United States is one of the world leaders in publicly and privately funded AIDS research, the United States has a poor record in AIDS-related public education. Virtually all European nations have spent far more money, per capita, on AIDS education than has the United States. Many dedicated individuals are working within different branches of the U.S. government, but in many ways their hands are tied.

Several demonstrations of civil disobedience have been used to prompt government action. No doubt additional actions will become part of the public debate.

The United States is still a young country. Its youth is reflected in the manner public health and social issues are handled. In any society, some individuals are more successful than others. In any society, some percentage of the population will not receive adequate nurturing or education, and these individuals are less likely to become socially productive.

In the United States, the consensus is that the nonproductive members are failures and that their situation is their own fault. In older western societies, the government assumes responsibility for these people, with the viewpoint that society (of which the government is head) failed the individual by not providing a proper foundation. Those governments attempt to create environments which prevent disadvantaged people from harming themselves and the people around them. Mature governments blame themselves for failures to produce well-balanced citizens. Immature societies blame the victims. There is a danger that U.S. society will come to blame people who contract cancer for not eating right, exercising enough, or managing their stress properly. The possibility that these people drank water containing carcinogens (cancer-causing chemicals) as children may no longer be considered.

Certain populations of individuals in the United States have long been recognized as reservoirs of certain diseases. Unless the situation drastically changes,

Figure 2: Government Resources

Description	Contact
National AIDS Hotline. 24 hour service. Government sponsored hotline. Keeps nation-wide list of AIDS-service organizations, physicians, test sites, support groups, local AIDS hotlines. Pamphlet on request.	1-800-342-7514
U.S. Conference of Mayors. A national organization composed of officials from cities hav-ing populations over 30,000. Interest areas are transportation, housing, human develop-ment and health. Its AIDS program serves as an information exchange for public officials. Backlogged with information requests, responses to public officials receive priority. The U.S. Conference of Mayors also distributes grants to community-based organizations for AIDS education projects.	**Grant Program:** (202) 293-7330 Mr. Richard D. Johnson Assistant Executive Director 1620 I Street, NW Washington, DC 20006
U.S. Dept. of Health and Human Services (HHS). HHS is the umbrella organization for several government agencies dealing with health and welfare, including the U.S. Public Health Service. The principal agencies involved in AIDS-related research and/or educa-tion are listed below, all belonging to the U.S. Public Health Service.	**AIDS Education Coordinator:** Shellie Lengel (301) 443-0292 5600 Fishers Lane Room 9–46 Rockville, MD 20857 **Assistant To Media:** Mary White (202) 245-6867 200 Independence Ave SW H.H. Humphrey Building Washington, DC 20201 General Info: (202) 475-0257
Centers for Disease Control (CDC). The CDC performs epidemiological study and sur-veillance of disease, mortality and morbidity; develops and conducts programs for dis-ease prevention; develops and conducts programs for training health care workers; pro-motes occupational health. List of national AIDS resources available.	**AIDS Referral Desk** (404) 329-3534 **STD Area** (404) 329-2552 **General Info:** (404) 329-3311 Centers for Disease Control 1600 Clifton Roads, NE Atlanta, GA 30329
National Institutes of Health (NIH). Composed of a number of institutes, the NIH con-ducts research within its own laboratories; funds research projects both in the United States and overseas; supports training for promising new researchers; and communicates research results to other researchers, scientists, and the public. Within NIH, the National Institute of Allergy and Infectious Diseases (NIAID) is the principle agency concerned with AIDS, funding research programs in drug therapy and vaccine development.	**NIAID Office** **of Communications:** (301) 496-5717 NIAID Room 7A-32 9000 Rockville Pike Bethesda, MD 20892

Alcohol, Drug Abuse, and Mental Health Administration. Seeking to control and prevent alcohol and drug abuse, and to prevent and treat mental illness, this agency conducts research in its own laboratories and supports outside research as well. Information is released through clearinghouses:	**Food and Drug Administration (FDA).** The FDA is a regulatory agency, responsible for keeping the nation's food and drugs "pure and wholesome." The FDA approves drugs after an application and testing procedure. Applicants conduct experimentation at their own expense after the FDA approves the testing procedure. In AIDS-related research, the FDA focuses on drug therapy and vaccine development.	**Health Resources and Services Administration.** Working with national and local organizations, this agency oversees the distribution and utilization of health care resources to the medically underserved populations and other groups with special needs. It provides funds and grants to organizations providing care for HIV-related illnesses and for AIDS-related education of health care professionals.
National Clearinghouse for Alcohol and Drug Abuse: (301) 468-2600 P.O. Box 2345 Rockville, MD 20852 **National Clearinghouse for Mental Health:** (301) 443-4515 Room 15C-05 5600 Fishers Lane Rockville, MD 20857	**Office of Consumer Affairs:** (301) 443-3170 5600 Fishers Lane Room 16-85 Rockville, MD 10857 **Office of Public Affairs: (Media Inquiries)** (301) 443-4177 5600 Fishers Lane Room 15-05 Rockville, MD 10857	**Office of Special Projects:** Dr. Samuel Matheny, Director (301) 443-6745 5600 Fishers Lane Room 14-43 Rockville, MD 20857

these populations, such as IV drug users, will continue to be the center of rapid HIV transmission and will continue to serve as a reservoir for the AIDS virus. IV drug users and deprived people who cannot afford health care already serve as reservoirs for tuberculosis and hepatitis B.

European nations and their treatment of socioeconomically disadvantaged people are examples for the United States. However, unless a drastic change occurs in American mythology or some courageous political and public health officials take a stand, the U.S. situation will not improve.

2. A Virus — The Invader

Structure and Function

A virus is a very, very small organism (every living thing is an organism). The average Human Immunodeficiency Virus (HIV) is about 0.000031 inches (100 nanometers) long. Tens of thousands of them could fit into the period at the end of this sentence.

Viruses are hard to find. An electron microscope, which can fill a small room, must be used to see them. But before using the microscope, one must first know where to look. Chemical tests of body tissues usually reveal viral chemical activity and, thus, the site of viral infection.

Viruses are responsible for many diseases, such as the common cold, the flu, and some childhood illnesses, such as mumps and chickenpox. Smallpox, yellow fever, and certain other deadly diseases are also caused by viruses. In some animals, viruses have been found to cause cancers, such as leukemia in cats. Some cancers in humans may also be caused by viruses.

Viruses are not cells. Cells are the structural units of most living things. Some organisms, like the amoeba, are one-celled organisms. Others, like humans, are multi-celled organisms. Cells contain fluid and specialized structures held together by an outer membrane. Cells reproduce by dividing in half. One cell divides to make two identical cells. Unlike cells, viruses contain no fluid nor do they perform any life processes such as growth or reproduction on their own. Instead, viruses infect (live in) the cells of other organisms. By some definitions of life, viruses are not really alive.

Viruses are parasites. A parasite is an organism that lives on or in another organism—called the host—and uses the host's chemicals and nutrients to live and reproduce. Being so small and able to use their hosts' nutrients, viruses survive as very simple physical structures. A virus consists of a strand or strands of DNA (deoxyribonucleic acid) or a strand or strands of RNA (ribonucleic acid) surrounded by a coat of protein. Most viruses have DNA cores. The Human Immunodeficiency Virus (HIV), however, has an RNA core.

Most living things—animals, plants, microorganisms, and even most known viruses—contain complete instructions for building and running the organism in DNA, the "master molecule." It is composed of four chemical building blocks, called *nucleotides*, which are like letters of the alphabet. Strung together in different combinations, they form a biological equivalent of words, sentences, and books.

Within a limited number of viruses, RNA, rather than DNA, is the carrier of information. To illustrate how RNA accomplishes this task, it is easier to first look at a human cell. Within human cells, DNA makes RNA. A chemical structure "reads" a string of DNA and, using a similar nucleotide alphabet, "writes" a strand of RNA. This process is called *transcription*, another word for writing.

While DNA stays in the center of the cell, the RNA travels around within the cell, building and running the cell, and making other chemicals which do most of the work.

The nucleotide alphabet is basically the same in all living things. A virus uses its host's alphabetical chemicals to write copies of itself. To do this, the virus hijacks the host cell. A typical DNA virus first latches on to the outside of a host cell, then injects its DNA strand into the host cell, leaving the protein coat outside. The viral DNA strand travels to the center of the host cell and splices itself into the host's DNA strand or strands. The hijacked host cell begins to make copies of the viral DNA. The host cell also makes proteins for the coat of the virus, creating additional hijackers to invade new host cells. This whole process is called *viral replication*.

In most RNA viruses, the RNA directly controls hijacking and replication in the host cell. However, HIV is different. Once injected into the host cell, the RNA strand of HIV writes dual strands of viral DNA. This backward writing is called *reverse transcription*. These newly written DNA strands then go on to hijack the cell and oversee the production of new RNA replicas. Reverse-writing viruses, like HIV, are called *retroviruses*.

In HIV, an enzyme called *reverse-transcriptase* (RT) performs the reverse transcription process. Enzymes are chemical workhorses. Human cells do not contain RT because they only write and have no need to reverse-write. Thus reverse transcriptase is virus-specific and an important target for anti-viral drug therapy.

Mutations and HIV

A mutation is a mistake, happening when some nucleotide word or phrase is misspelled. Either a letter or word is left out or put in the wrong place or an extra letter or word is added. A mutation is not an intentional act on the part of an organism. Most mutants are not strong organisms, and many of them simply die.

For example, suppose this page contained an error in spelling (a mutation). What are the chances that this error would (1) improve the book, (2) make the book worse, or (3) make no difference? In most instances, a mistake makes the book worse. The same is true for organisms. However, a small, almost unnoticeable mistake may lead to the development of a new strain.

Since a single virus may make hundreds of replicas, a few mistakes here and there make little difference. Even if many mutants die, replicas are, in biological terms, cheap to make. If 1 or 2 of 1000 mutants get written instructions that enable them to survive better than their fellows in the existing environment, then these organisms produce replicas of themselves which may, in time, become new strains of the virus.

Recent evidence suggests that HIV mutates at a rate five times faster than the influenza (flu) virus, an extremely rapid rate compared to most known viruses. This exceptional rate of mutation has important implications for HIV detection, treatment, and vaccine development, which are discussed later.

Figure 3: The Human Immunodeficiency Virus

Name	Chemical Structure	Desig-nation	Description
1. Envelope Protein	Glycoprotein	gp120	The protein coat, or envelope, of the virus is composed of globes of this protein. (These globes sit on thin sticks of the transmembrane protein.)
2. Trans-membrane Protein	Glycoprotein	gp41	These sticks of protein support the globes of the envelope protein; the resulting unit resembles a lollipop. This protein is anchored in the membrane of the virus.
3. Mem-brane	Lipid (fat)		The membrane of the virus is actually a portion of membrane stolen from the host cell and altered for HIV's use—not a substance manufactured by the virus.
4. Core Protein	Protein	p24	Several proteins form the viral core. The core proteins seem tightly bound to the virus's RNA core.
5. RNA Core	Ribonucleic acid	RNA	Two stands of RNA, coiled together, form the cylindrical core. Packed into the core are several molecules of reverse transcriptase (RT).

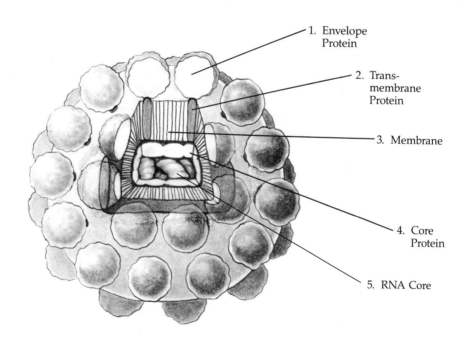

1. Envelope Protein
2. Trans-membrane Protein
3. Membrane
4. Core Protein
5. RNA Core

Figure 3: The Human Immunodeficiency Virus (HIV)—an artist's rendition. Its two RNA strands, containing genetic information, are condensed into a cylinder-shaped core and coated by layers of protein and lipid (fat). This illustration is not to scale. On an actual virus, a vast array of tiny "lollipops" coats the virus's surface, forming a "solid" layer which obscures the underlying structures.

Figure 4: HIV Genes

Name	Product	Description
ENV	gp160, gp120, gp41	Contains instructions for making glycoprotein 160. Gp160 splits to form envelope (gp120) and transmembrane (gp41) proteins. Gp160, gp120, and gp41 are antigenic. The gp 160 and gp 120 gene products have been generated by genetically-engineered yeast, bacteria, insect, and mammalian cells in several laboratories.
GAG	p55, p24, p18	Creates proteins of HIV's core. The gene p55 cleaves into p24 and p18. Most lentiviruses have similarity in their gag region. P24 and p18 are antigenic.
POL	Reverse Transcriptase (RT)	Reverse transcriptase is the enzyme which reverse-transcribes the viral RNA into viral DNA. RT, necessary for viral replication, is unique to viruses. Two RT's may exist, having different molecular weights. Most lentiviruses have similarity in their *pol* region. RT is antigenic.
TAT (ORF S)	*Trans*-acting (RT)	This protein helps regulate protein replication by triggering or speeding up the replication process. Without this protein, HIV is not potent.
ART (ORF)	Not identified	Called the "fast forward" gene. Sits side by side with *tat*, like twin engines. Both genes function as on-off switches. *Art* is anti-repression factor. Also seems to affect *gag* and *env* gene expression.
SOR (ORF Q)	Protein—function not identified	Creates protein found in infected cells. This gene is not necessary for HIV to replicate or kill cells.
ORF F (3'ORF)	Protein—function not identified	Protein product is antigenic. This gene is not necessary for HIV to replicate or kill cells.
R	Unidentified	The R gene product is found in infected cells. Little is known of its character and its function is not yet recognized.

Notes: Typical lentivirus genes are: gag, pol, env, tat. ORF stands for "open reading frame." Roughly speaking, an open reading frame is a strand of nucleotides that is "shared" by a couple of genes. The numbers gp160, gp120, etc., refer to the molecular weight of the protein molecules. These molecules also vary in weight, according to the strain. For example, the envelope protein ranges from 110,000 to 120,000 daltons in different isolates. A dalton is a unit of molecular weight.

Genes

Thus far, scientists have found eight *genes* on the RNA strand of HIV. Genes are like complete chapters in an organism's book of life. Each gene contains the complete instructions for making one protein or chemical. The word "genetic" refers to genes or the information they contain. In comparison, humans have approximately 100,000 genes.

Compared to most known retroviruses, which have two to three genes, HIV is a large retrovirus with complex genetic organization. Not all of HIV's genes and gene products have recognized functions. Figure 4 lists the recognized HIV genes and their functions.

Two genes of HIV are of particular interest because these two genes mutate rapidly. These genes are the *env* and the *tat,* discussed in detail below. The other genes of HIV do not appear to change much. Together or separately, these two highly variable genes may determine the virulence (deadliness) of this virus in its human hosts. The existence of different HIV strains of varying virulence may explain why some people infected with HIV die rapidly while others survive without serious ill effects for long periods of time. This explanation for HIV's apparently varying virulence is still theory. A number of other factors discussed later may determine viral virulence or host susceptibility to HIV.

Env. Embedded in the nucleotide segment of the *env* gene are the instructions for building HIV's protein coat, or envelope. If this gene mutates, the mutant virus which results, if it survives, is likely to have an altered protein coat. Since the human immune system recognizes viral invaders by their protein coats, new mutants may be able to hide from the human immune system, gaining time to replicate and infect more host cells. Although up to twelve different HIV strains, all thought to evolve from a common ancestor, have been found within the same person, this theoretical hiding procedure is probably not, by itself, the cause of immune system failure in AIDS.

HIV's protein envelope protects the RNA core and determines which cells HIV is able to infect. Projecting from the viral coat are small protein structures called *epitopes.* These projections serve as keys which unlock membranes of the host cells, allowing HIV to inject its RNA strand into the cell. Epitopes are highly specific, meaning they fit into the host cell's "locks" exactly, just as house keys and car keys are highly specific. Viruses are able to bind to locks of only one or a small number of cells. These locks, called *receptor sites,* normally allow cells to communicate with each other, either by direct contact or via communicating chemicals.

Since the *env* gene is constantly mutating through mistakes made during replication, individual viruses with slightly varying epitopes are constantly being released into the host. Most of these mutants do not survive. Some variants, however, may unlock host cells better than other variants. Theoretically, such HIV variants could overwhelm and kill host organisms faster than variants that are less effective at receptor site binding. Alternatively, the epitopes of viral mutants may be able to unlock the membranes of new cell types, providing the virus with a new population of cells to infect.

Tat. The *tat* gene produces a small protein called the *trans*-activating protein, which the virus uses to trigger its replication process inside the host cell. Since the instructions written into the *tat* gene are highly variable, the protein product is also highly variable and may also determine virulence. Some forms of the activating protein may be more effective in triggering replication than others. Thus, some strains of HIV may replicate at a faster rate than others, again, overwhelming the host faster than other strains.

Differences in HIV Strains

During viral epidemics, the overall number of viruses infecting a host population greatly increases. As more viruses replicate, more mutants are produced, and the likelihood of the development of new strains increases.

The flu virus, an RNA virus, is an example of a rapidly mutating virus, which is a nuisance to humans. Each winter new strains return to infect us. The HIV retrovirus has the potential to develop many new strains, both because of its high mutation rate, and because the virus has been shown to replicate very rapidly. This rapid rate of replication may be one of the reasons why the virus is so dangerous.

For a virus, diversity—having different strains—is an advantage. New strains may be able to infect new types of cells within the same host or infect new types of host organisms. Diversity also protects the virus from destruction by the host's immune system. Out of several mutant strains, perhaps at least one will survive the continuing attack of the host's immune system.

Different strains of HIV exist. The line between one HIV strain and another is indistinct. One way to differentiate strains is to chemically examine the genetic codes and to arrange the strains according to the spelling of their nucleotide sequences. This extremely difficult, time-consuming, and expensive procedure is performed on very few HIV isolates. The more common ways to differentiate strains are to examine external structure(s) or to observe life processes within the host or in the laboratory. Experiments show that some HIV strains differ in replication rates.

First, laboratory experiments show that HIV isolates taken from seriously ill patients replicate faster than HIV isolates taken from patients who have not become seriously ill over time. To isolate a virus means to take it from where it grows in the host and to grow it in a laboratory dish. Isolates taken from two people may or may not be different strains.

Second, HIV infects several cell types, but the two of importance in these studies are T-cells and macrophages. (See Chapter 3.) HIV isolated from T-cells replicate better in T-cells than in macrophages. HIV isolated from macrophages replicate better in macrophages than in T-cells. These isolates may or may not highlight the abilities of distinct strains. Some other factor(s) may be involved.

These experiments are *in vitro*, (in glass) experiments. Biological events rarely occur *in vitro* as they do *in vivo*, (in a living being). When discussing biological experiments, it is important to distinguish between the two types of experimentation.

Figure 5: The Name Game

Acronym	Description	Also Known As
ARV	AIDS-Related Virus.	HIV, HTLV-III, LAV
HIV-1	Human Immunodeficiency Virus 1. HIV-1 been isolated from patients in the United States, Europe, and Central Africa and is considered to be the cause of AIDS. The AIDS cases found in South America, the Carribean, and scattered around the world are also currently thought to be caused by HIV-1.	ARV, HTLV-III, LAV-1
HIV-2	Human Immunodeficiency Virus 2. HIV-2 may be renamed soon. Some isolates called HIV-2 cause AIDS or AIDS-like diseases while others do not. HIV-2 and HIV-1 have been found co-infecting European patients. HTLV-IV is also classified as HIV-2, however HTLV-IV may not cause illness. HIV-2 has core proteins similar to HIV-1, but its envelope proteins are different. The ELISA blood test for HIV-1 does not detect HIV-2.	HTLV-IV, LAV-2
HTLV-III	Human T-cell Lymphotropic Virus-III The name originally given the virus by American researchers.	ARV, HIV, LAV
HTLV-IV	Human T-cell Lymphotropic Virus-IV HTLV-IV found originally in healthy West Africans. Now thought more closely related to a monkey virus than to HIV.	HIV-2
LAV	Lymphadenopathy-Associated Virus. The name originally given the virus by French researchers.	ARV, HIV, HTLV-III

Discovery of various HIV isolates receives much media acclaim in the United States. Some of these discoveries are important, but some, in time, may prove to be not HIV, but other viruses having similar structures or traits, or other viruses which contaminated the lab equipment. Figure 5 lists some of these isolates and characteristics. In time, scientists will uncover more strains of HIV and continue adding to our knowledge.

The Family of Retroviruses

HIV belongs to the family of viruses called *Retroviridae,* or retroviruses. As a group, retroviruses can live in their hosts for a long time without causing any sign of illness. This is called *viral persistence.* In most animals, retrovirus infections last for life. Retroviruses are not very tough: they die when exposed to heat, alcohol, and most common disinfectants, and usually do not survive if the tissue or blood they are living in dries up. Retroviruses have high rates of mutation and, as a result, tend to evolve very quickly into new strains. HIV seems to share these traits with other retroviruses.

Recent research has allowed scientists to classify HIV more specifically within the retrovirus family. HIV is now classifed as a lentivirus. Lentiviruses are one of the three subgroups of Retroviridae. Before the appearance of HIV, lentiviruses were known to infect only the ungulate (hoofed) animals, such as domestic sheep, goats, cattle, and horses. (See Figure 6.)

Scientists initially classified HIV as a lentivirus based on its morphology (structure) and its biologic properties (internal functions, life patterns, and effects on hosts). Later, HIV's nucleotide sequences were compared to the genes of the visna (sheep) virus. The visna virus was found to share the HIV's complexity of genetic organization and to have similar genes. The researchers concluded that the two viruses had a relatively recent common ancestor, firmly placing HIV in the lentivirus family.

Figure 6: Other Lentiviruses

Equine infectious anemia virus (EIAV). A virus causing anemia in horses. Anemia is a loss of blood cells. Some of the antibodies to EIAV cross react with HTLV-III.

Caprine arthritis-encephalitis virus (CEAV). A virus infecting goats. Arthritis is an inflammation of a joint. Encephalitis is an inflammation of the brain.

Ovine maedi-visna virus (MVV). Also known as the visna virus. Causes fatal encephalitis in sheep. It has several "conserved" nucleotide regions reminiscent of HIV, and the antibodies to MVV cross react with the core proteins of LAV.

Other Lentiviral Diseases

Ovine pulmonary ademomatosis. A chronic lung disease of sheep characterized by cancerous glandular growth. Lungs fill with mucous and mucous-secreting cells.

Cattle lymphocytosis. Recently recognized disease. Lymphocytosis is an abnormal increase in the number of lymphocytes.

The visna virus is now being used as an animal model of AIDS. The visna virus, found in sheep, causes a slowly progressive neurological disease. Like HIV, the visna virus infects brain tissue, is slowly progressive, and uses macrophages as "Trojan horses" to enter the brain. The visna virus, and its progression of disease in sheep, in some circumstances, is now viewed as a comparison model for HIV infection. In sheep herds, visna virus is considered to be 100 percent fatal within 15 years. Effective drugs against the visna virus have never been developed for sheep. Slaughter is more cost-effective.

3. Humans — The Host

Several cell types in the human body serve as homes for HIV. Most of these cells are parts of the body's *immune system.* The immune system defends the body from disease. It is composed of a number of specialized cells, several organs, and a group of biologically active chemicals. The human immune system is like a wall which protects us from armies of germs. This wall can be compared to a jigsaw puzzle — many parts fit together to form a solid surface. If pieces are missing or damaged, germs rush in through the holes. This happens with AIDS.

Over most of the body, the skin prevents germs from entering the body. Thus, germs can enter only through some body opening, cut, or wound. Once inside the body, germs trigger an *immune response.* All cells belonging to the body have special molecules on them that are like flags with the word "friend" on them. The cells of the immune system try to destroy anything present in the body that is not carrying a friendly flag, anything that is "nonself." Any substance or object that triggers the creation of antibodies is called an *antigen.* Antigens may be whole germs, parts of germs, or some germ product. Antibodies are discussed below.

Once inside a cell, any virus usually harms its host. Forced to manufacture viral replicas, the host cell neglects its own life processes. Gradually, like a machine wearing out, the host cell starts to fail and dies. In truth, the best thing a virus can find is a host cell that does not break down and that can produce replicas indefinitely. In a biological time frame, parasites are often very deadly to new host organisms. If a new parasite strain is too deadly, it kills its host before other hosts are infected, and the strain dies out. Over biological time, successful parasites and their new hosts learn to accommodate each other.

T-Cells

Once in the body, HIV replicates well in a group of white blood cells called the *lymphocytes,* or T-cells for short. Among the T-cells, the T4-cell is HIV's favorite; that is, HIV easily infects and replicates in the T4-lymphocyte. Figure 7 illustrates the life cycle of HIV in the T4-cell.

The T4-lymphocyte, also called the "helper T-cell," performs a vital job in the immune system. It locates germ invaders by circulating through the bloodstream and bumping into them. After recognizing an invader, T4-cells release chemical alarms which trigger other parts of the immune system into action against the invader. In response, lymphocytes and other immune cells rapidly grow in number. Some of these cells are cytotoxic (cell-killing) and directly attack the invader. Some are lymphocytes which keep sounding the alarm to draw other cells into the area. The T4-cell recognizes only viral, fungal, and parasitic invaders and triggers only those portions of the immune system that act against these invaders.

Another lymphocyte infected by HIV is the T8-lymphocyte, or suppressor

25

T-cell. T8-cells balance the action of T4-helpers by secreting chemicals to block the effects of the T4-cell's alarms. Together, T4-cells and T8-cells regulate the body's immune response to invaders. Also, T8-cells help the immune system recognize (and not attack) the cells of its own body.

T-Cell Function and HIV

Once HIV hijacks a T-cell the lymphocyte stops functioning well, although this change is not immediately apparent. HIV's takeover is a quiet event. The virus's RNA reverse transcribes its DNA partner, then—nothing happens. Evidently, very little or no viral replication takes place until the host T-cell is activated by some antigen. Then, instead of functioning normally, the T-cell manufactures the invader's viral RNA strands. The activating antigen does not seem to be another HIV but some unrelated viral, fungal, or parasitic invader.

The "opportunistic diseases" common in AIDS prove malfunction in the T4-cell population. The opportunistic diseases seen in AIDS are caused primarily by fungi, viruses, and parasites, many of which we encounter daily. Some of these organisms live permanently in our bodies, although in healthy people they are held in check by the correctly functioning immune system.

HIV infection seems to kill T-cells. So in addition to poor T-cell performance, the actual number of T4-helper cells in an infected person decreases. How HIV kills cells is not clear. Many other viruses fill the host cell with viral replicas, causing the cell to burst open: destroying the cell by spilling its contents out along with the new viruses. This event is called *lysis*. T-cell lysis is not the cause of T-cell death with HIV as once thought. The loss of T-cell function, leading to cell death, seems related to a gradual buildup of viral DNA and RNA strands within the infected cell.

Some T8-suppressor cells also die during HIV infection. As a result, the immune system is not properly suppressed in some infected patients and they have an auto-immune response, meaning that parts of their immune system attack their own bodies.

Macrophages

HIV is able to infect and replicate well in macrophages. Macrophages are large white blood cells which engulf and digest invaders. Macrophages do not have receptor site locks similar to T-cells, so HIV does not enter the cell that way. It is possible that HIV is eaten by the macrophage and hijacks the cell from inside.

Macrophages are called *monocytes* when they are circulating in the blood. Monocytes change into various types of macrophages (with different names) in order to perform search-and-destroy missions within tissues of the lung, brain, and interstitial (tissues connecting the organs) regions. Despite the name changes, all forms of macrophages basically work the same way: they eat things. Some macrophages travel around within the body, others become attached to one spot, eating what comes by.

Macrophages are often the first scouts of the immune system to encounter invaders, particularly in the area of a cut or wound. After engulfing the invader, the macrophage makes copies of the invader's epitopes and displays them on

Figure 7: HIV Life Cycle in Host Cell

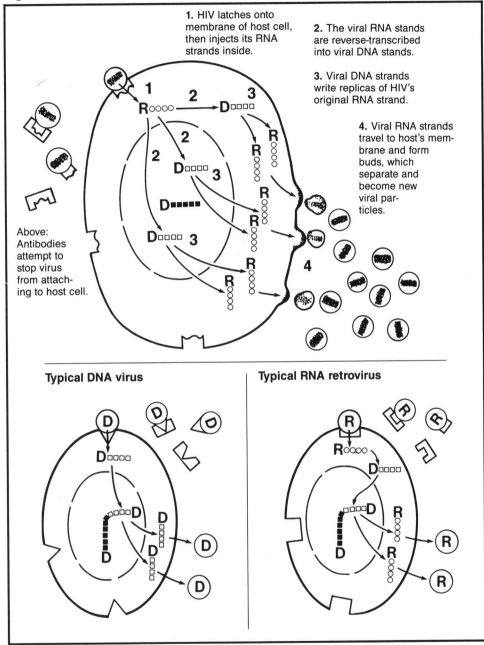

1. HIV latches onto membrane of host cell, then injects its RNA strands inside.

2. The viral RNA stands are reverse-transcribed into viral DNA stands.

3. Viral DNA strands write replicas of HIV's original RNA strand.

4. Viral RNA strands travel to host's membrane and form buds, which separate and become new viral particles.

Above: Antibodies attempt to stop virus from attaching to host cell.

Typical DNA virus

Typical RNA retrovirus

Figure 7: Schematic diagrams of viral replication. HIV replicates more rapidly than most known viruses, perhaps because of the free-floating DNA strands it creates. Most viruses attach their DNA strands to the host's DNA before viral replicas are made.

its own cell membrane. These copies of the invader epitopes sit right next to the "friend" flags. In effect, the macrophage makes a "wanted poster" of this new invader. The macrophage then travels about showing the wanted poster to T4-helper cells, which triggers the T-cells into action. Macrophages also release chemicals which stimulate both T-cell and macrophage production and draw macrophages and lymphocytes to the site of infection.

HIV infection does not seem to kill macrophages. In some infected human patients, HIV appears to change monocyte function slightly, not affecting the ability to engulf invaders, but affecting the release of communication chemicals. In HIV-infected macrophages, the transformation from monocyte to another of its specialized forms, seems to be the trigger of viral replication. Macrophages can produce high levels of virus for a long time in laboratory conditions.

In vivo (in living beings) macrophages may play an important role in spreading HIV infection in the body, both to other cells and to HIV's target organs. First, HIV quietly spreads from macrophage to macrophage before any other cells of the immune system notice. Second, macrophages, in their different forms, travel to the brain, the lungs, the bone marrow (tissue in the hollow centers of some bones), and to various immune organs, and bring HIV along with them.

HIV's ability to infect brain tissue is particularly important. The brain and the cerebral spinal fluid (CSF) are vulnerable sites, and, consequently, are specially protected sites. CSF cushions the brain and the spinal cord from sudden and jarring movements. The *brain-blood barrier*, a chemical phenomenon, normally stops foreign substances from entering the brain and the CSF. Unfortunately, HIV-infected monocytes can slip past this barrier. For HIV, macrophages may be Trojan horses, enabling HIV to enter the immune-fortified domain of the central nervous system—the brain, the spine, and all nerves. Once in brain tissue, monocytes change into microglial cells. In addition to acting as an immune system scout, microglial cells may make a number of regulatory molecules that balance immune system function and perhaps other functional systems.

HIV isolates taken from macrophages seem to grow better in macrophages than in lymphocytes. In human experiments HIV isolates taken from lymphocytes seem to grow better in lymphocytes than in macrophages. These peculiarities of replication rates may be evidence of distinct HIV strains.

B-Cells

According to laboratory evidence, HIV may infect B-cells, another type of lymphocyte. B-cells, triggered by the chemical alarm of T4-cells, rapidly grow in number and manufacture millions of antibodies, discussed in detail in the next section. It is possible that B-cells can be activated directly by virus antigens; the evidence is not yet conclusive.

The epitopes of HIV do not fit the membrane receptor site locks of B-cells, so it appears that HIV cannot normally enter and infect B-cells. However, in laboratory experiments, HIV is able to infect B-cells, if the B-cells are first infected by the Epstein-Barr virus, which is the cause of infectious mononucleosis. The Epstein-Barr virus appears to change B-cells in some way, allowing subsequent HIV infection. Whether similar events occur in humans is not known, but the evidence suggests that B-cells might serve as reservoirs of HIV or as viral replication sites.

B-cells function almost normally in most infected patients. Small defects in B-cell functions exist, seemingly resulting from the disrupted communication with other cells, not from some internal B-cell defect. HIV can grow and replicate within B-cells transformed by the Epstein-Barr virus, without destroying the host cell.

Antibodies

Antibodies are proteins which stop invaders. Antibodies prevent viruses from attaching to the membrane, or outer covering, of the host cell. Viruses and antibodies fit together like pieces of a puzzle. Antibody molecules physically and chemically fit the molecules in the virus's protein coat. New antibodies must be tailored for each new invader. Figure 7 illustrates how antibodies work.

B-cells make antibodies and release them into the bloodstream. After being triggered by antigens or the T4-cell alarm, B-cells multiply and manufacture tailor-made antibodies to stop the new invader.

After an antibody and virus join, they are eaten by macrophages or cleared from the blood by the liver and spleen. Some B-cells become *memory cells* which are stored by the immune system. Memory cells remember the antibodies they have created. If the same virus ever gets into the bloodstream again, these cells rapidly begin antibody production. However, if the virus has mutated, as the flu does in its yearly journey around the world, the old antibodies cannot stop it. New antibodies must be created to neutralize the new mutant virus. While this antibody production is taking place, the viral invader has time to multiply and gain a foothold, and the infected person suffers the symptoms of the flu.

Antibodies and HIV

The human body makes anti-HIV antibodies, but they apparently do not work effectively. The anti-HIV antibody works against HIV in a laboratory dish, but things rarely occur in life the same way they do in the laboratory.

In several experiments where HIV has been isolated from blood, large numbers of anti-HIV antibodies were also found. This indicates that, even though the anti-HIV antibody is present, it has difficulty latching onto the virus, and, therefore, provides little protection.

The human body creates antibodies directed against a number of HIV proteins, namely the envelope proteins (gp120), the transmembrane protein (gp41), and the proteins of HIV's core (p24).

Antibodies cannot enter blood cells. An antibody can only attack viruses in the plasma. Plasma is the fluid part of the blood and does not include the blood cells. Once inside a host cell, HIV has nothing to fear. Cells can generate anti-viral chemicals within themselves, but these too seem ineffective against HIV.

Once a virus gets inside the host cell, it is likely to remain there for the rest of the host's life unless some other anti-viral mechanism within the body, or some artificial chemical is able to destroy the virus or the infected cell.

Other Sites of Infection

Laboratory experiments show that HIV can replicate in a wide range of human cells if injected into the cells artificially. HIV's difficulty is in entering cells. HIV's epitopes, the protein projections on the protein coat, successfully unlock the membrane of lymphocytes, but not the membranes of most other cells. So HIV infects only the cells it can enter. However, researchers are finding that this includes more cells than previously thought.

HIV is found to directly infect tissues of the *brain,* but it seems to infect nerve cells only rarely. HIV seems marginally able to infect various connective tissues in the brain and apparently does not replicate well in them. In the brain, HIV infection seems to be located in macrophages and microglial cells. Again, macrophages probably introduce HIV into the brain and central nervous system.

The symptoms of brain infection are forgetfulness, impaired speech, tremors, and seizures, and in some cases personality change and dementia (deterioration of mental state due to physical damage).

HIV may also infect cells of the *retina,* part of the eye. The retina is nervous tissue located at the back of the eyeball. The retina can be considered as an extension of the brain.

HIV nests in the tissues of bone marrow. *Bone marrow* is found in the hollow centers of long thin bones. Both T-cells and B-cells are born in the bone marrow. B-cells mature in the bone marrow, while T-cells travel to the thymus to mature. Thus T-cells and B-cells may become infected with HIV at birth. Initially, macrophages probably carry HIV to the bone marrow in their travels.

The *thymus* is an organ of the immune system which lies behind the breastbone. It stores lymphocytes while they mature and stimulates them with a chemical. Initial evidence suggests that HIV infects the epithelium (skin) cells of the thymus, possibly infecting T-cells at that site and interfering with the chemical maturation of lymphocytes.

HIV seems to be able to infect cells in the *lung,* but only in children so far. HIV infection does not occur within the lungs as pneumonias do; rather HIV seems to infect the interstitial cells, the connective tissue at the site. Macrophages evidently carry HIV to the lungs.

In laboratory experiments, HIV infected cells of both the *rectum* and the *colon.* The colon is basically the large intestine, and the rectum is the lowest portion of the large intestine, directly before the anus. The ability of HIV to infect these cells means HIV may be transmitted via anal intercourse more easily than previously thought.

Animals, Too?

The Human Immunodeficiency Virus (HIV) has not been isolated from any animal other than humans.

Besides HIV, other viruses cause immunodeficiency, and other viruses are lymphotropic (like to grow in lymphocytes). Certain animal viruses having these traits were discovered during the early days of the AIDS epidemic. Perhaps rather inappropriately, animal researchers created names for these new viruses that suggested that these viruses are linked to AIDS and to HIV. By doing so, these researchers prompted media coverage of their research projects, and, in addition, greatly contributed to the confusion.

This section and Figure 8 survey these other viruses in an effort to eliminate this confusion.

The Rhesus Monkey. The rhesus monkey, or rhesus macaques (*Macaca mulatta*), native to Asia, is commonly used in medical experimentation. They are relatively easy to breed, inexpensive to maintain, and are useful replacements for humans for certain biological functions. The U.S. government sponsors four regional primate research centers which keep sizeable populations of rhesus macaques.

Reportedly, around 1976, immunodeficiency disease and lymphomas (cancers) were noticed in captive rhesus monkeys at the California Primate Research Center. The problem gradually appeared at the other government-sponsored primate research facilities in Massachusetts, Washington, and Oregon. This disease is not AIDS; its symptoms are different, but these researchers named this disease "SAIDS," for "simian *a*cquired *i*mmunodeficiency *dis*ease." *Simian* means "relating to an ape or monkey."

Researchers eventually isolated a virus thought to cause SAIDS and, predictably, named it the "SAIDS-Related Virus," or SRV for short. The discovery of SRV-2, another isolate, soon followed.

It is now known that SRV is not related to HIV at all; it is a different type of virus. SRV is related to the Mason-Pfiser Monkey Virus (MPMV), a well-known monkey virus which causes immunodeficiency.

Because SRV would not always induce SAIDS when injected into macaques, researchers kept looking for other viruses and eventually isolated another one which caused immunodeficiency in macaques. This virus was named STLV-III, short for "Simian T-cell Lymphotropic Virus-III." STLV-III is now classified as a lentivirus; but again, it is not HIV.

When HTLV-III was renamed HIV, STLV-III followed the naming convention and was renamed SIV, the Simian Immunodeficiency Virus. Since SIV has been found in other species of monkeys, the SIV found in rhesus macaques is labeled SIVmac. SIVmac causes disease in macaques, but this immunodeficiency is not AIDS.

The African Green Monkey. The African green monkey (*Cercopithecus aethiops*) is native to Africa. Soon after SIV (STLV-III) was discovered, antibodies to SIV were discovered in wild African green monkeys, prompting media reports that the AIDS virus was found in African monkeys. Again, SIV is not HIV.

Eventually, SIV was isolated from African green monkeys and labeled SIVagm. SIVagm does not cause disease in African green monkeys. Recent studies of antibody cross-reactivity reveals that SIVmac and SIVagm are not closely related. These antigenic tests reveal SIVagm to be more closely related to HTLV-IV, the nonpathogenic virus found in humans of western Africa. In addition, recent nucleotide sequencing studies suggest that SIVagm originated in humans as HTLV-IV or something similar and then spread to monkeys.

The Sooty Mangabey Monkey. The sooty mangabey monkey (*Cercoebus atys*)

Figure 8: Monkey Viruses

Name	Description
SRV	SAIDS-related virus. SAIDS stands for "simian acquired immunodeficiency syndrome." SAIDS is not equivalent to human AIDS. SRV is not related to the Human Immunodeficiency Virus (HIV). SRV causes immunodeficiency in captive rhesus monkeys. It is related to the the Mason-Pfizer Monkey Virus (MPMV), a well-known monkey virus, which also causes immunodeficiency in rhesus macaques. Existing isolates are SRV-1 and SRV-2
SIV	Simian Immunodeficiency Virus. Also called STLV-III. SIV is not the Human Immunodeficiency Virus (HIV). It is closely related to HTLV-IV. HTLV-IV is found in humans but does not cause disease. Historical genetic data suggests that humans were the orginial reservoir of HTLV-IV, which spread to monkeys and evolved into SIV. SIV was first isolated from captive rhesus macaque monkeys, then isolated from two other types of monkeys. At this time, SIV is tentatively classified as a lentivirus. Antibodies of SIV core proteins cross-react with core proteins of HIV-1 and HIV-2. Antibodies to SIV's envelope cross-react only with HTLV-IV envelope proteins.
SIVmac	The SIV isolated from captive rhesus macaque monkeys in the United States. Causes immunodeficiency in captive Rhesus Macaque Monkeys. Macaques are native to Asia.
SIVagm	The SIV isolated from African Green Monkeys. Does not cause illness in African Green Monkeys.
SIVsm	The SIV isolated from (African) Sooty Mangabeys Monkeys. Does not cause illness in Sooty Mangabey Monkeys.
STLV-III	Simian T-cell Lymphotropic Virus. Also known as SIV.

is native to Africa. Recently, SIV was discovered in this monkey and named SIVsm. SIVsm does not cause disease in sooty mangabeys, but reportedly induces disease when injected into macaques. According to antigenic tests SIVsm is not closely related to HIV. It is more closely related to SIVmac than to SIVagm or HIV.

Summary

Many different viruses have similar protein coats and similar physical structures. When using antigenic tests to differentiate these viruses, mistakes are likely to happen.

For example, HTLV-III was orginally thought to be a close cousin of HTLV-I and HTLV-II, the human T-cell *leukemia* viruses. In early research it seemed that the antibodies of HTLV-I and HTLV-II reacted strongly with the HTLV-III antigen. With further research, it was found that HTLV-III was not closely related to the leukemia viruses at all. Consequently, the "L" in HTLV-III evolved from a meaning of leukemia to lymphotropic.

The same problem is evident with SIVagm and HIV. Using antibody tests, monkey SIV antibodies reacted with HIV. As a result, SIV was called the AIDS virus. Recent research has shown that although SIV anti-core antibodies react with HIV's core proteins, the anti-envelope antibodies of SIV do not latch onto the envelope proteins of HIV. The cores are similar, the protein coats are different; therefore the viruses are different.

This research implies that SIV and HIV, similar at the core, have taken different evolutionary pathways and developed different epitope keys to unlock different host cells—HIV for human lymphocytes and SIV for monkey lymphocytes. Literally, this is how families grow. Every virus, every organism, has evolutionary cousins.

The discovery of SIV in rhesus macaques is important as an animal model of AIDS, a living laboratory for studying immunodeficiency, viruses, and drugs. Rhesus monkeys and SIV are a biological parallel to humans and HIV.

HIV has been injected into a number of apes and monkeys, and only the chimpanzee shows signs of illness. However, the chimpanzee does not catch AIDS, only lymphadenopathy, a milder form of HIV infection.

4. Characteristics
of HIV Infection (AIDS)

As with many infectious diseases, response to HIV infection varies. A person's susceptibility to infection may vary according to the person's genetic (inherited) makeup, the site of inoculation (where the virus entered the body), the presence of other infectious diseases, the person's history of infectious diseases, the strength of the particular strain, and the condition of the person's health. What is known about these cofactors will be discussed later.

Most symptoms, diseases, and abnormal physical conditions related to HIV infection are listed in Figure 10 and Figure 11. Since AIDS is a syndrome, the presence of these symptoms, diseases, and conditions varies from one patient to another. The diseases may occur in sequence (one after another) or simultaneously.

Since HIV infection is often a slowly progressive syndrome, it has been necessary to construct systems for identifying and classifying its various forms or stages. Defining the forms of HIV infection or types of AIDS is a difficult task, due both to the variable forms of HIV infection and to the changing medical understanding of AIDS. Consequently, several different AIDS classifications exist, fulfilling the various needs of their creators.

The Popular Classification System

The popular classification system is the collection of haphazard definitions that evolved as the AIDS epidemic unfolded. They are presented here because (1) they are easy to understand, and (2) they are widely used by the media. However, other classification systems exist.

By popular definition, four different forms of HIV infection exist. Beginning with the mildest form, they are: (1) the healthy carrier state, (2) lymphadenopathy syndrome (LAS or LAN), (3) AIDS-related complex (ARC), and (4) AIDS. So far, not everybody infected with HIV has come down with AIDS. Many HIV-infected people have remained healthy for years. Others have developed stable lymphadenopathy or ARC. As time passes, however, many people progress to a worse disease state. In some HIV-infected people, the different forms of infection represent the progressive stages of the disease. Some HIV-infected people experience a feverish, flu-like illness soon after they become infected. The symptoms of this illness are discussed in Chapter 6.

Healthy Carrier State. A *carrier* is someone who is infected with a disease and shows no clinical symptoms but who is capable of infecting other people with the disease.

HIV has been isolated from healthy people who show no clinical signs of HIV infection. Also, antibodies for HIV have been detected in healthy individuals. The presence of antibodies could mean the successful destruction of the virus by the person's antibodies. Some people who have anti-HIV antibodies may go on to develop LAS, ARC, or AIDS.

A small study suggests that HIV-infected people become more infectious (able to infect others) over time. It is not yet clear when an HIV-infected person becomes infectious. At this time, the only safe practice is to assume that anyone carrying the virus is capable of transmitting it to others. For specific information, see Chapter 5.

Lymphadenopathy Syndrome (LAS or LAN). *Lymphadenopathy* means "disease of the lymphatic system." The lymphatic system is the human body's second fluid system and contains a clear fluid called *lymph*. (See Figure 9.)

The lymphatic system is a vital part of the body's immune system. The lymphatic system aids the blood system by draining fluid out of the body's tissues. It is not a closed loop like the bloodstream, meaning it does not flow in a circle, and it has no pump like the heart. Nevertheless, lymph flows from smaller vessels into the larger lymph ducts located in the upper chest. In doing so, lymphatic fluid passes through a series of filtering stations called *lymph nodes,* or *lymph glands.*

Lymph nodes filter bacteria, foreign substances such as antigens, and dead white blood cells from the fluid. In each lymph node, a variety of compartments contain T-cells, B-cells, and macrophages. T-cells can migrate back and forth between the blood system and the lymphatic system, perhaps introducing HIV into the thymus. Thus all the factors need for an immune response are brought together in lymph nodes. With all this activity, lymph nodes often swell during infection. This nodal swelling is why doctors feel the lymph nodes around the neck, under the armpits, and in the groin during physical checkups. A healthy lymphatic system is required for an effective immune system.

One of the key signs of lymphadenopathy is swollen lymph nodes. Of course, any infection, such as the flu, causes the lymph nodes to swell. Nodal swelling caused by the flu and most other infectious illnesses passes relatively quickly, as the other symptoms of illness fade. However, with HIV infection, the lymph nodes remain swollen for months, with no other signs of a related, temporary infectious disease. Consequently, lymphadenopathy is sometimes called *persistent generalized lymphadenopathy* (PGL).

Stable cases of lymphadenopathy have been directly related to HIV infection. Lymphadenopathy is not in itself life-threatening, although a portion of the cases will advance into ARC or AIDS.

AIDS-Related Complex (ARC). AIDS-related complex is a more serious level of HIV infection. The symptoms generally include the symptoms of lymphadenopathy, plus one or two abnormal body conditions revealed by laboratory tests or the presence of one or more opportunistic infections.

Laboratory tests can determine whether the number of T4-cells in the patient has dropped in relation to the number of T8-cells. This decrease in the number of T4-cells sometimes can be detected during lymphadenopathy. In addition in ARC, skin usually exhibits *anergy* to antigens, meaning the skin fails to develop allergic reactions such as swelling, itching, and redness, after being pricked by antigen-covered needles. Some patients have opportunistic infections even though their skin still displays allergic inflammations.

ARC is the level of HIV infection where some differences between HIV-infected people are seen and where a prognosis (prediction about the progression of the disease) might be ventured. On average, patients with Kaposi's sarcoma, a skin cancer, as their first clinical sign of disease, excepting LAS, survive longer than patients whose first clinical sign is some opportunistic infection. Some researchers say ARC patients with Kaposi's sarcoma are more comparable to LAS patients than to other ARC patients.

Immune system differences exist between patients with Kaposi's sarcoma and patients with opportunistic infections. Those with opportunistic infections average lower numbers of T4-cells and their T-cells are not able to grow and divide as well in response to antigens.

Acquired Immune Deficiency Syndrome (AIDS). AIDS is the full-blown syndrome. Again, not all possible symptoms, conditions, or opportunistic infections appear in any one patient. Figures 10 and 11 list the diseases and conditions common to AIDS patients. The diseases developed because of immune

Figure 9: Lymphatic System

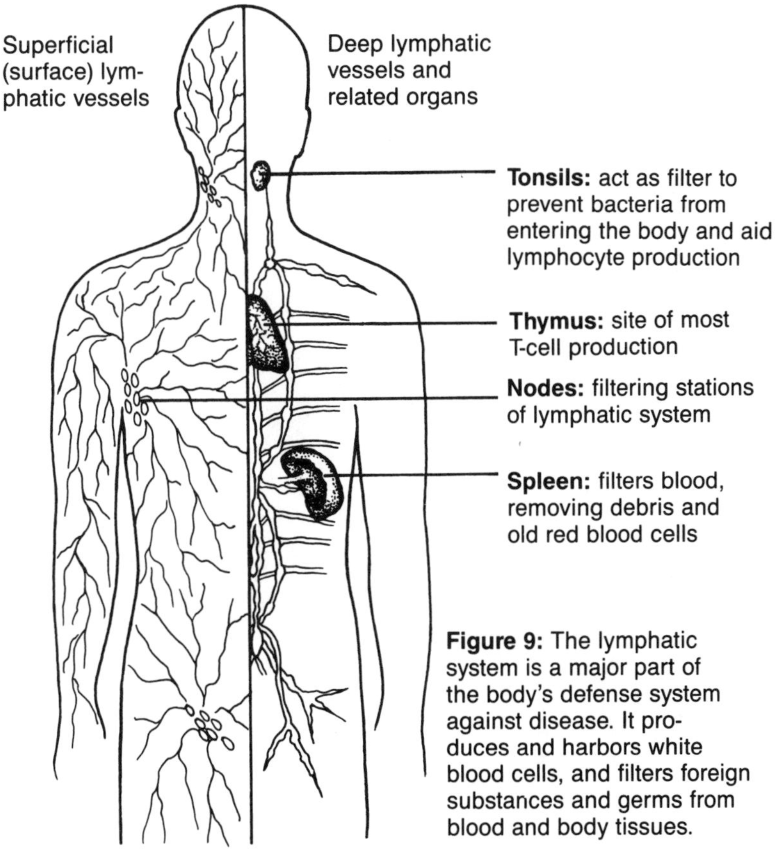

Superficial (surface) lymphatic vessels

Deep lymphatic vessels and related organs

Tonsils: act as filter to prevent bacteria from entering the body and aid lymphocyte production

Thymus: site of most T-cell production

Nodes: filtering stations of lymphatic system

Spleen: filters blood, removing debris and old red blood cells

Figure 9: The lymphatic system is a major part of the body's defense system against disease. It produces and harbors white blood cells, and filters foreign substances and germs from blood and body tissues.

Figure 10: Diseases Common to AIDS

Protozoa
Pneumocystis carinii Pneumonia (PCP). Caused by *Pneumocystis carinii*, common world wide. Infects lungs. Previously found in kidney transplant patients whose immune system had been chemically suppressed. Occurs in 60% to 80% of U.S. AIDS patients. Initially responsible for 30% to 50% of deaths among AIDS patients, now brought under better control. Mortality probably decreased by early diagnosis. *Diagnosis:* Microscopic examination of tissue removed from bronchi, the breathing tubes leading to the lungs, or sputum. Sometimes chest X-rays, lung function tests, blood tests, etc. Lung biopsy, surgical removal of lung tissue, was common but now thought by many not to be worth the risk of surgical infection. *Treatment:* Responds to chemical therapy. Persistent—relapses after treatment ends. Suppressive therapy now being attempted.
Toxoplasmosis. Caused by *Toxoplasmosa gondii*. Infects blood and many tissues. In AIDS patients, tendency to infect central nervous system causing encephalitis or brain abcess. Also causes pneumonias and hepatitis. Common to humans, many domestic and wild animals, and birds. Humans may catch it from droppings of cats, birds, and from undercooked meat, especially mutton. *Diagnosis:* CAT scan or brain biopsy. *Treatment:* Chemical therapy. Reoccurs after treatment ends, thus treatment required indefinitely.
Cryptosporidiosis. An enteritis (inflammation of the intestines) caused by *Cryptosporidia muris* and/or *C. difficile*. Causes severe cramping and diarrhea. One-celled parasite common to domestic and wild animals. Many minor, non-life-threatening outbreaks occur in day-care centers. In AIDS patients, may be a major cause of mortality. *Diagnosis:* Chemical testing of stool sample. *Treatment:* Effective treatment is difficult in immunosuppressed patients. Experimental drugs being tested.
Isosporiasis. Caused by *Isospora belli*, commonly found in the small intestine of humans. Causes enteritis. *Diagnosis:* Stool sample. *Treatment:* Infection seems to repond to therapy.
Strongyloidiasis. Caused by species of *Strongyloidea*, roundworm parasites found in small intestines of mammals. Can infect lungs by inhalation or enter body through mucous membranes; organism then migrates to intestines. Can infect central nervous system. Present in feces and contaminated soil. At certain stage larvae can penetrate skin. *Diagnosis:* Stool sample. *Treatment:* Difficult in immunocompromised patient.

Fungi
Cryptococcosis. Caused by *Cryptococcus neoformans*, a fungus found in pigeon manure. Common among humans, and other mammals, especially cats. Inhaled in dust, it infects skin and lungs. Causes pneumonia in rare instances, most often causes meningitis (inflammation of membranes lining the spinal cord and brain membranes). Also causes endocarditis (inflammation of membranes lining the heart); and skin ulcers. *Diagnosis:* Usually by culture of infected tissues or substances.

Treatment: Responds to treatment and sometimes managed by suppressive therapy.

Aspergillosis. Caused by species of *Asperigillus,* some species normal residents of humans. Infects lungs and the mucous membranes of the ear, nose and throat. Also causes endocarditis, meningitis, and skin lesions. May be widespread throughout body.
Diagnosis: Culture of sputum, mouth, or stool.
Treatment: Responds to treatment. Persistent.

Candidiasis. Caused by *Candida albicans,* a fungus common to skin, mouth, vagina, and gastrointestinal tract of humans. In HIV-infected patients, often takes form of white spots or patches on sides of tongue, perhaps on mucous membranes on inside of cheeks, and commonly lodges under nailbeds and the skin around the armpits, groin, and rectum. Sometimes affects lungs. May be first clinical sign of HIV infection.
Diagnosis: Examination of organisms swabbed from mouth.
Treatment: Often responds to treatment and sometimes managable. Indefinite treatment may be required.

Histoplasmosis. Caused by *Histoplasma capsulatum* and/or *H. duboisii,* fungi contracted by breathing fungal spores in soil dust. Common to AIDS patients in Europe and Africa, rare in the United States. Usually infects lungs, sometimes is disseminated throughout body.
Diagnosis: Culture of sputum or infected tissues.
Treatment: Standard antibiotics have been used. Little information available.

Blastomycosis. Caused by *Blastomyces dermatitidis,* a fungi usually found in soil. Usually infects lungs first, then disseminates to the central nervous system, the kidneys, and sites in the skin.
Diagnosis: Culture of infected tissues.
Treatment: Some response with standard antibiotics, little information available.

Viruses

Cytomegalovirus (CMV). Normally present in the salivary glands of humans. In AIDS patients it is often widely scattered throughout the body. Suspected in promoting appearance of Kaposi's sarcoma. Causes problems in eyes, colon, lungs, liver, and adrenal glands. With the relative success of PCP treatment, cytomegalovirus is now considered the major cause of mortality.
Cytomegalovirus is frequently spread in day-care centers, where it has been shown to survive on toys for 30 minutes and on plexiglass for 8 hours. It can be shed in urine.
Diagnosis: Tissue biopsy and culture.
Treatment: Therapy is still experimental.

Herpes simplex infections. Caused by herpes simplex viruses 1 (cold sores on lips) and 2 (sores on genitals). Commonly forms small, painful blisters from time to time at chosen location. In HIV-infected patients it forms chronic ulcer, often affecting the face, and sometimes the eyes. Anal area often affected in homosexual males.
Diagnosis: Clinical recognition or culture.
Treatment: Responds to treatment, recurs frequently.

Figure 10: Diseases Common to AIDS (Continued)

Herpes Zoster. Caused by varicella-zoster virus, another herpes virus, which causes shingles and chickenpox. Virus may remain latent for years. Seems limited to humans. Causes inflammation of spinal and cranial ganglia (nerve roots). Painful blisters form on the skin, usually following the nerve path along the face or neck. Herpes zoster is common among people not infected with HIV. Often an initial clinical sign in AIDS patients. Can also be disseminated throughout body.

Diagnosis: Clinical recognition or culture.

Treatment: Treat for pain. Experimental drug treatments.

Epstein-Barr. The Epstein-Barr virus (EBV) is the suspected cause of mononucleosis and some lymphomas. Epstein-Barr is implicated as a co-factor in a number of other diseases and auto-immune conditions. EBV is thought to disrupt immune system regulation by disrupting T-cell function. In AIDS patients it causes oral hairy leukoplakia, fuzzy white spots on the tongue which do not rub off as does the "hairy tongue" caused by smoking. Also suspected of causing B-cell lymphomas, the rapid unregulated multiplication of B-cells, and interstitial pneumonitis, the inflammation of connective tissue of lungs. Possibly EBV lies latent until HIV infection occurs.

Diagnosis: Blood tests.

Treatment: Experimental treatments.

Bacterial

Mycobacterium infection. Caused by *Mycobacterium avium-intracellulare*, a bacterium commonly found in human saliva. Causes a type of tuberculosis in humans, producing lesions in the lungs. Disseminated, it causes problems in the intestines, blood, liver, and spleen.

Diagnosis: Culture of blood or stool.

Treatment: Treatment not very effective.

Tuberculosis (TB). Caused by *Mycobacterium tuberculosis*, a non-opportunistic infection common to non-HIV-infected people. Infects the lungs, disseminated in some AIDS patients. A major killer in the past, social hygiene education and effective medical treatment eliminated TB from most of the Western world, except for poor populations lacking access to medical care. Contracted by inhalation of infected droplets.

Diagnosis: Culture of sputum.

Treatment: Antibiotics. Difficult in immuno-compromised patients.

Salmonellosis. Caused by species of *Salmonella*, bacteria which are the common cause of "food poisoning" in spoiled meat. Common among many types of mammals. Present in unpasteurized milk and milk products—items to be avoided by HIV-infected people.

Diagnosis: Culture of stool.

Treatment: Difficult in immunosuppressed patients.

Syphilis. Recently discovered via autopsy in a high percentage of AIDS patients, though only a small number of cadavers were examined. While not detected in AIDS patients by standard procedures, the organism causing syphilis initially infects the genital organs (or other site of exposure) and eventually may infect the brain and nervous system, gradually causing dementia and insanity. Syphilis is a non-opportunistic disease, easily contracted by healthy people.

Diagnosis: Blood tests, biopsy of sores, test of cerebrospinal fluid.

Treatment: In non-AIDS patients, effectively treated.

Nocardiosis. Caused by *Nocaria asteroides*, bacteria primarily infecting the lungs, which spread to the central nervous system causing abscesses in the brain, skin, and other areas.

Diagnosis: Examination of infected tissue or culture.

Treatment: Difficult in immunocompromised patients.

Shigellosis. Caused by species of *Shigella*, some species normally found in the intestines of humans. Causes severe diarrhea in AIDS patients.

Diagnosis: Examination of culture or infected tissues.

Treatment: Standard antibiotics attempted.

Haemophilus influenzae. Bacteria responsible for respiratory tract infections, also the common cause of conjunctivitis ("red eye").

Diagnosis: Examination of culture or infected tissues.

Treatment: Standard antibiotics have been used.

Cancers

Kaposi's sarcoma (KS). Malignant skin cancer. Previous to its appearance in AIDS patients, "classical" Kaposi's sarcoma was only found in old men of Mediterranean background or in Africa. Classical Kaposi's sarcoma progresses slowly, requiring years to spread over the skin. "Epidemic" Kaposi's sarcoma, seen in AIDS patients, often appears in small splotches and grows rapidly, affecting the skin, lungs, gastrointestinal tract, genitals, and other organs. Occurs as first clinical symptom in approximately 40% of homosexual patients, while rare in heterosexual IV drug users. Onset may be encouraged by "poppers" (amyl or butyl nitrite). Conversely, factors promoting the development of Kaposi's sarcoma may be transmitted sexually, while poppers are only a marker of high sexual activity. Cytomegalovirus (CMV) is thought to have a role, since CMV is found in Kaposi's sarcoma biopsy specimens.

Diagnosis: Clinical recognition.

Treatment: Drug treatment, radiation, immune modulators. Persistent, but treatment sometimes improves patient's condition.

Lymphomas. Lymphoma is a term used for the cancerous growth of tissue in the lymphatic system. In AIDS, lymphomas are common in the lymphatic tissue of the brain, bone marrow, intestines, rectum, and subcutaneous sites. Hodgkin's disease—lymphoma of the spleen, liver and other tissues—is sometimes reported in AIDS patients. Burkitt's disease, a form of malignant lymphoma normally found only in African children, is also infrequently reported in AIDS patients. Lymphomas in AIDS are suspected to result from the unregulated multiplication of B-cells inside lymph nodes. The Epstein-Barr virus is suspected of causing B-cell lymphomas in and out of HIV-infected people.

Diagnosis: Clinical recognition or tissue biopsy.

Treatment: Drug treatment, radiation, immune modulators.

system failure. Drug treatments are available for many of these opportunistic infections, but without the support of a healthy immune system, the drugs fail to cure the diseases fully. These opportunistic diseases, curable under other circumstances, are the causes of death for most AIDS patients. In this book, individuals having full-blown AIDS will be called AIDS patients. All other HIV-infected individuals will be designated as "HIV-infected."

Other Classification Systems

The Centers for Disease Control (CDC) created an epidemiological classification system. *Epidemiology* is the study of disease in populations. In addition, CDC established the surveillance definition of AIDS.

Classification and definition are two different things. The CDC classification system, like the popular system discussed above, attempts to describe the stages of HIV infection. Historically, the CDC classification system has focused on the clinical presentations of AIDS, that is, the appearance of opportunistic diseases and AIDS-related conditions.

The CDC surveillance definition is used by doctors reporting AIDS to government recording stations. It is used to count AIDS patients. Therefore, the AIDS cases reported by CDC, and subsequently by the media, refer only to CDC-defined AIDS, which is similar to full-blown AIDS of the popular classification. An abbreviated version of the "CDC Surveillance Case Definition for Acquired Immunodeficiency Syndrome" is in Appendix A. This new definition, effective September 1, 1987, will increase the total number of AIDS cases by 10 to 15 percent, as more HIV-infected people will fall under the AIDS classification.

According to a small 1985 study, an estimated 11 percent of AIDS cases are not reported because of breakdown in reporting procedure (usually absence of patient by time diagnosis is made).

The CDC surveillance definition of AIDS is, in a sense, the legal definition of AIDS and is necessarily the focus of much criticism. A number of HIV-infected people who were very sick did not match the original CDC definition of AIDS. These individuals either did not display the necessary symptoms to match the CDC definition or exhibited conditions which excluded them from this definition. Unfortunately, some dying HIV-infected individuals were denied financial, social, and medical support services set aside for AIDS patients because they did not officially have AIDS. CDC continually updates its definitions and classifications, most recently in early Fall 1987, when they were considerably broadened.

A number of other classification systems have been developed by researchers experimenting with drug treatments. In these classifications, the absolute number of T4-cells in the blood usually is used to measure disease progression. A patient's T-cell count is a better indicator of actual health status than clinically visible symptoms. Also, the T-cell count gives a numerical basis for determining the effectiveness of a drug or treatment.

Neurological (Nerve) Disorders

AIDS is primarily known as a disease of the immune system. However, AIDS is now recognized as a disease of the central nervous system, too. The central nervous system consists of the brain, the spinal cord, and the nerves. The term *neurologic* means "related to the central nervous system."

The common neurologic problems found in HIV infection are: (1) dementia, the loss of thinking functions due to physical brain damage; (2) myelopathy, a disease of the spinal cord; and (3) peripheral neuropathy, a disease of the nerves, which usually affects motor (movement) skills in AIDS. In AIDS, death from brain damage can occur without any other clinical signs. AIDS-related behavior changes and psychiatric problems are discussed in Chapter 9.

Initial neurologic symptoms are generally mild, but steadily grow worse, sometimes accelerating abruptly in the latter stages. On occasion, serious neurologic problems develop within a few days. About 10 percent of all AIDS patients exhibit neurological symptoms as the first sign of AIDS. An estimated 50 percent of all AIDS patients eventually develop clinically evident neurologic disorders.

Quick recognition of neurologic symptoms in AIDS is difficult because the early signs of neurologic disorder are similar to the symptoms of emotional depression. Depression is basically a sadness so strong that it interferes with a person's ability to function in society. Most AIDS patients and HIV-infected people become extremely depressed at some point in the course of their illness.

Initially, doctors and researchers thought opportunistic infections were solely responsible for dementia in AIDS. However, it was discovered that HIV, carried into the central nervous system by macrophages, grows in various brain tissues and causes damage on its own. In 100 autopsies, direct HIV infection of brain tissue was found in over half. In general, autopsies revealed a greater degree of brain damage from both HIV and opportunistic infections than was suspected from the patient's clinical appearance.

Cryptococcus and *toxoplasmosis* are the most frequent opportunistic organisms found in the brain. One may be more common than the other depending on geographic region. These organisms form large colonies, primarily in the white matter and subcortical structures of the brain, with relative sparing of the cortex. There is some suspicion of viral activity in the hypothalamus. *Mycobacterium* has also been isolated from brain tissue but does not seem to form colonies. Undiagnosed *syphilis* infection of the brain has recently been seen as a problem. Syphilis is a sexually transmitted disease which initially infects tissues in the sex organs but can spread quietly and unnoticed into the central nervous system. Syphilis is not considered to be an opportunistic infection, since it is able to infect humans without the help of HIV. Lymphomas are another problem in the central nervous system. (See Figure 11.)

Weight Loss

Weight loss is a major sign of advanced HIV infection. This weight loss and accompanying malnutrition may pave the road for opportunistic infections and substantially contribute to patient death.

Figure 11: Physical Disorders Common to AIDS

Anergy. Anergy is the lack of skin response (inflammation, itching, redness) to common allergens. Allergens are simply things that cause an allergic response. Allergic responses often include antibody production. Many HIV-infected people lose their ability to react to common laboratory allergens. This condition is also called delayed hypersensitivity.

Autoimmune Response. In some AIDS patients, the patient's immune system seems to attack the patient. This autoimmune response may be responsible for the depletion of various types of blood cells because the immune system may be indiscriminately destroying both infected and non-infected blood cells.

Blindness/Deafness. Blindness results from damage done to the eyes by opportunisitic infections. Deafness seems caused by nerve damage caused either by HIV or opportunistic infections of the central nervous system.

Blood Disorders. AIDS patients seem to have abnormal coagulation responses, such as blood clotting and scab formation, as demonstrated in one study. Also, AIDS patients often show lack of one or another type of blood cells, perhaps due to cell-killing autoimmune response or cell death induced by HIV infection. Blood disorders include: lymphopenia, the lack of lymphocytes (white blood cells that engulf germs); lack of blood platelets; and anemia, the lack of red blood cells.

Body Composition. In AIDS patients, the composition of the body undergoes notable changes. Body fat content drops. Intracellular (inside cell) water volume decreases, accompanied by relative increase in extracellular (outside cell) water volume. Potassium levels, important for nerve and muscle cell function, drop.

Cardiac dysfunction. Sometimes heart dysfunction is the cause of death in AIDS, perhaps resulting from damage of lymphomas, Kaposi's sarcoma, or opportunistic infections. Stenosis, the narrowing of the cardiac valves is reportedly common.

Diarrhea, Malnutrition & Wasting. Diarrhea is frequently severe and life-threatening among AIDS patients, leading to "wasting," serious weight loss. Malnutrition can adversely affect immune response.

Hyperplasia. Excessive growth of normal cells in an organ.

Kidney dysfunction. Kidney failure sometimes occurs. Early in the AIDS epidemic, the presence of kidney problems excluded a person from having "AIDS" as defined by the Centers for Disease Control.

Paralysis. Resulting from damage to central nervous system or peripheral nervous system by HIV or opportunistic infection.

Severe diarrhea is one contributory factor in weight loss, particularly in some disease-advanced patients. Diarrhea can swiftly threaten death by draining the body of fluids and necessary minerals.

In HIV infection, the cause of weight loss that is not due to diarrhea is not yet known. Factors at work may include: (1) simple *starvation* from inadequate food, perhaps due to loss of appetite and oral disease problems; (2) *malabsorption,* where food intake is adequate but cannot be absorbed, perhaps due to Kaposi's sarcoma or *Cryptosporidia* in the intestines; or (3) altered metabolism, which interferes with the use of nutrients by the cells.

Malnutrition harms the immune system. It is known to cause lymphopenia (lack of lymphocytes), decreased macrophage activity, and it may impair immune cell growth and multiplication in response to an antigen. Malnutrition also leads to organ dysfunction and prevents recovery from opportunistic infections that might otherwise be non-life-threatening.

Progression of HIV Infection

The great mystery of HIV infection is why some people rapidly progress to AIDS, while others seem to stabilize at the stages of LAS or ARC without symptoms.

In the first years of the AIDS epidemic (and the AIDS epidemic is still young), only 2 to 3 percent of HIV-infected people developed AIDS, while another 20 percent or so developed LAS and ARC.

Now it seems that a greater percentage of infected people progress into serious illnesses. These percentages vary from study to study. In one reasonably sized study of HIV-infected people, 36 percent developed AIDS and a total of 62 percent developed clinical symptoms over an estimated 6 years of infection. People seldom know at what point in time infection occurred.

Differing predictions for AIDS patients can now be made, depending on which clinical symptoms first appear in the patient.

The appearance of Kaposi's sarcoma alone as the first clinical symptom of AIDS infection has the most favorable prognosis. Those patients live an average of 21 months after diagnosis.

A person who developed *Pneumocystis carinii* pneumonia as the first clinical symptom of HIV infection lives an average of 12 to 13 months after diagnosis. Patients with other opportunistic infections survive an average of 11 months. Patients who have both Kaposi's sarcoma and *Pneumocystis carinii* as initial symptoms survived an average of only 6 to 7 months.

These average rates of survival are really windows into the past. They reveal the mortality situation as it was in the first 5 or 6 years of the AIDS epidemic. With limited advances in treatment, mortality rates should change somewhat, although life may not be pleasant. In truth, the AIDS epidemic is still too young for the full story of HIV infection to be told.

The mortality of AIDS varies from population to population. For example, homosexual males in New York City have higher AIDS mortality rates than homosexual males in Washington, D.C. Both groups have higher mortality compared to homosexual males in Denmark. On limited evidence, it seems that fewer hemophiliacs develop clinical symptoms than either homosexual males or IV

Figure 12: Markers of Progression

Small, measurable, biological changes in HIV-infected patients may act as red flags, signalling imminent progression of HIV infection. The information offered here is tentative, based on small scale medical research experiments, not on large scale epidemiological study.
Antibodies. The antibody directed against proteins in the virus's core (anti-p24) is found in the early stages of HIV infection. If the levels of anti-core antibody in the blood decrease, this seems to indicate a progression of the HIV infection. This fall in levels of anti-core antibodies seems to happen before the T4-cell count drops (thus before opportunistic infections occur), and, according to one theory, marks a stage of rapid destruction of T-cells by HIV.   The anti-envelope (anti-gp120) antibody is also a marker. High blood levels of anti-gp120 combined with high levels of anti-cytomegalovirus antibodies seem to indicate an ARC person will soon advance into AIDS, at least in homosexual males.   Anti-lymphocyte antibodies may be detectable in the blood before any clincial symptoms develop. Anti-lymphocyte antibodies, which attack infected lymphocytes in the host, are found in HIV-infected people. These anti-lymphocyte antibodies may be, in part, responsible for the destruction of uninfected T4-cells, and numerous other red and white blood cells.
Beta-2-Microglobulin. Microglobulin is a molecule found on the surface of most cells. This molecule is associated with the "self" markers on cells, the "friendly" flags. "Beta-2" refers to how the molecule acts in certain laboratory tests.   Microglobulin can be detected and measured in urine. Rising urine levels indicate an increase in cell destruction, possibly meaning that HIV is rapidly replicating and destroying many cells. See neopterin.
Herpes Zoster. The presence of herpes zoster infections, a common infection among HIV-infected people, may indicate marked depression of immunity. The degree of pain and the severity of zoster seem related to future progression to more serious illness.
Interferon. Interferon is a chemical that cells produce to prevent viral replication. Several types of interferon exist. Two of them are thought to be markers of disease progression: alpha-interferon and gamma-interferon. Both are measurable in the blood.   It seems HIV-infected people who are not able to generate gamma-interferon in response to laboratory antigens are at high risk for developing an opportunistic infection within a year.   Alpha-interferon also undergoes changes. It apparently becomes more acid-liable as HIV infection progresses; the clinical importance of this is not clear.
Neopterin. Neopterin can be measured in the urine. Roughly speaking, neopterin is a break-down product of the building blocks used in making RNA and DNA. An increase in urine levels may indicate increased viral activity in the body.   Patients with confirmed AIDS/ARC were found to have raised levels of B-microglobulin and neopterin levels. These two substances may be earliest markers of HIV infection, in absence of other clinical and biological markers. The levels of these substances seem to rise approximately at the same time as antibodies become detectable in the blood, before T- cell count falls.

46

Prolactin Levels. Prolactin is a hormone produced by the hypothalamus, an organ considered to be part of the brain.

During HIV infection, the blood levels of prolactin increase, perhaps indicating viral activity in the hypothalamus. It seems levels of prolactin can change before other immunological changes occur.

Life processes under partial hypothalamic control include body balances of water, sugars, fats, hormones, and body temperature. The hypothalamus controls the autonomic ("automatic") nervous system, which controls the involuntary muscles, the muscles used without thinking, like breathing muscles. The hypothalamus may also affect mood and motivational behavior.

T-Cell Levels. Perhaps the best measure of disease progression is the absolute number of T4-cells. The lower the T4-cell count, the sicker the person.

The measurement of T-cells proliferative ability is a second way to detect disease progression. Proliferation is the ability of T-cells to grow and multiply when stimulated by an antigen. Decreasing proliferative ability represents a progression in HIV-infection.

drug users. Infection of hemophiliacs occurred relatively recently in the AIDS epidemic. Time was required for HIV to find its way into the blood products necessary to hemophiliacs.

The differences in infection and mortality rates may be due to availability or lack of quality medical services, regional lifestyles, personal lifestyles, presence of other diseases, or the presence of different strains of HIV, and so on.

Apparently, some people can fight HIV infection on their own. In some cases, HIV-infected people developed antibodies to HIV and experienced drops in their T4-cell count. Their T-cell counts became antibody free.

Also, small numbers of homosexual men with Kaposi's sarcoma have experienced spontaneous remission and remained clinically well for years. These people may or may not have had AIDS. In studies, homosexual males have tested positive for HIV initially and then become antibody-negative later. Possibly, the antibody tests were inaccurate.

A small percentage of seriously ill AIDS patients seem to hold on. If a person survives 3 years with full-blown AIDS, the mortality rate seems to level off. This might be a result of treatment.

AIDS in Children

HIV infection in children is a somewhat different matter. Children get fewer opportunistic diseases, but the syndrome progresses much more rapidly than in adults.

Most children with AIDS are newborns or infants who contracted HIV from their mothers. Most of these mothers were IV drug users or sexual partners of IV drug users. Other children contracted HIV infection from blood transfusions.

In HIV-infected newborns, clinical symptoms usually develop within 6 months of birth. Most HIV-infected newborns die within 2 years. Survival past 36 months is rare, but does occur.

For some infants, the damage from HIV infection begins in the womb. Many children born to HIV-infected mothers have small heads and diminished brain weight (microcephaly), abnormal distances between the eyes (ocular hypertelorism), upward or downward slanting eyes, short flattened noses, and prominent boxlike foreheads. Such children tend to be born prematurely and to be small for their age. HIV-infected infants often fail to thrive.

Less than one-quarter of all children with AIDS get the opportunistic infections found in adults. Kaposi's sarcoma is rare in children. Hepatitis B infection and B-cell lymphoma are less common in children than in infected adults. However, children have another set of problems.

Bacterial infection, including septicemia, which is the presence of many bacteria in the bloodstream, is a problem. Bacterial infection is the result of the inability of B-cells to fight bacteria by making anti-bacteria antibodies. This B-cell defect appears to occur much sooner in children than in adults, although it is also possible that infant B-cells are too immature to mount an antibody response.

Other problems of children include lymphadenopathy, enlargement of the spleen and liver, salivary gland enlargement, kidney problems, and perhaps destruction of the thymus. AIDS-related blood problems include loss of blood platelets, which interferes with blood coagulation and scab formation at wounds, and an excess or lack of antibodies.

HIV-infected children also have a unique lung condition called *lymphocytic interstitial pneumonia* (LIP), which occurs in the absence of other opportunistic lung infections. Interstitial tissue, in a sense, is connective tissue. HIV is not found in the bronchi, the tubes leading to the lungs, and the alveoli, the tiny air sacs of the lungs, as are the germs that cause pneumonia. Thus coughing is not likely to expel large numbers of viruses or virally infected cells. However, during interstitial lung infections, a suction action draws substances from the interstitial area into the bronchi, where these substances become enmeshed in mucus. Thus the presence of HIV in sputum is possible. Generally, overt ("visible") LIP is only observed in children having no other lung infections.

The neurologic symptoms of HIV-infection are most visible in older children. There is a delay or absence of most developmental milestones, particularly motor (movement) deficits in younger children and perceptual-motor deficits and speech problems in older children.

5. Catching AIDS

Most cases of HIV infection have been transmitted through sexual contact, intravenous drug use with HIV-contaminated needles, transfusions of blood and blood products, and passage of the virus from mother to child. This section describes confirmed and suspected methods of transmitting HIV.

The Mechanics of Transmission

In order for a person to become infected with HIV, the virus must travel from the inside of one person to the inside of another person, arriving with its RNA intact. Then the virus, or its intact RNA strands, must maneuver past whatever immune defenses the body has at the site of entry. Finally, the virus must insert its intact RNA strands into a host cell. Once inside a host cell, HIV's RNA strands can prepare for replication. After replication, replica viruses infect other host cells, either by circulating through the plasma (the fluid portion of the blood), or by attaching to new hosts when blood cells collide.

Generally, more than one virus enters the body at one time. More likely a person encounters dozens, hundreds, or thousands of viruses during exposure. The more viruses present, the better the chance that one or more succeeds in finding a host cell and replicating. So the concentration of viruses in a substance is an important factor in transmission. *Concentration* is the number of viruses per unit of volume.

Throughout most of the short history of AIDS, the scientific consensus has been that a person has to be immunodeficient (immune system not working well) in order to catch AIDS. Now it appears that HIV cannot enter a host cell unless the host cell is immune-activated, meaning the cell is already fighting some other infection. In the laboratory, at least, HIV cannot infect cells unless the cells are stimulated. Many of the people who now have AIDS, namely, homosexual males, IV drug users, and hemophiliacs, are thought to be constantly in a state of immune activation. See the sections concerning these individuals in Chapter 12.

Some evidence suggests that infected cells, rather than cell-free viruses passed from one person to another, are the major vehicles of HIV transmission. This is thought to be the case even though transmitted cells are attacked as foreign invaders inside another human. Infected cells may be present in any body substance or tissue containing lymphocytes or macrophages. Cell-free HIV has been found outside of cells in human plasma and semen, and may also exist in other body fluids and substances.

HIV's route of entry into the body may influence whether it successfully establishes infection or not. At a particular site of entry, a virus may not live long enough to successfully infect cells. Nor might there be many adequate host cells with the proper receptor sites (locks) near the site of entry. Also, the type and number of such nonspecific immune defenses as macrophages, natural killer cells, and nonspecific antibodies vary from location to location. Little is known about the effect of site of entry on risk of HIV infection.

Few things are constant in biology. Very likely the presence and concentration of the virus in various bodily substances changes over time, just as the ability of an HIV-infected person to infect other people probably changes over time. Current evidence suggests that a person becomes more infectious as HIV infection progresses. It is best to assume that all HIV-infected people are infectious during the entire course of their infection.

The Mucous Membranes. *Mucous membranes* are thin tissues which protect many openings and passages in the human body. These membranes secrete *mucus* which contains anti-germ chemicals and keeps the surrounding tissues moist. There are mucous membranes in the mouth, inside the eyelids, in the nose and air passages leading to the lungs, in the stomach, along the digestive tract, in the vagina, and in the anus.

The mucous membranes of the eyes and mouth are often doorways into our bodies for such highly infectious viruses as the flu. You can catch the flu from a person in the following manner: The person coughs in his or her hand, you shake hands soon afterward, and then your virus-carrying hand touches your mouth or eyes.

The danger with AIDS is totally different from that with influenza. First, the flu is highly infectious because the flu virus lives in the lungs, throat, and sinuses. Therefore, a high concentration of viruses is present in the sputum (the substance expelled by coughing or by clearing the throat). Second, coughing forces many viruses out of the lungs and into the air or into the sick person's hand or handkerchief. Third, the flu virus is definitely able to penetrate the mucous membrane.

With AIDS, the major infection sites are the bloodstream and the central nervous system. While HIV-carrying macrophages are found in the connective tissues of the lung and in oral and mucous membranes, the number of viruses present does not seem great. The virus is present in low concentrations, if at all, in saliva and sputum. So coughing should not expel a large quantity of viruses, if any.

Many viruses, if placed on the surface of a mucous membrane, can travel through the membrane and enter the tiny blood vessels inside. HIV does not seem to do this effectively, although at least two people seem to have contracted HIV infection from exposure of mucous membranes to infected blood. However, these people are the exception rather than the rule.

Where the Virus Is Found in Humans

HIV is found in any body fluid or substance which contains lymphocytes. Such substances include blood, saliva, semen, tears, mother's milk, vaginal secretions, urine, and feces.

Scientists have successfully isolated and cultured (grown) live HIV from some of these substances. Isolating and growing viruses is a difficult task; success is never guaranteed. The possible reasons for failure are many, including the scientist's skill in the laboratory, or his or her cleverness in creating a proper environment for viral growth. However, in or out of the human body, viruses are like flower seeds planted in a garden—some grow and some do not. Consequently, culturing viruses is not a sure way to test for their presence. The purpose of isolating and growing viruses is to prove that they exist—alive—in the substances tested. Live viruses can transmit disease. Virus cultures also provide scientists with living viruses to use in experiments.

When attempting to detect the presence of HIV for medical purposes, doctors test for the presence of the anti-HIV (usually gp120) antibody, which can be done quickly, cheaply, and with more accuracy. Antibodies, however, are found only in the blood.

Blood. Live HIV has been extracted and cultured from the blood of AIDS patients, ARC patients, LAS patients, and healthy HIV-infected individuals, some of whom later developed AIDS. Not every attempt to extract and grow HIV from AIDS patients has been successful. In fact, some researchers report more difficulty isolating the virus from the blood of AIDS patients than from the blood of ARC and healthier patients. There may actually be few HIV viruses present in the blood of AIDS patients because most of the host T4-cells have been destroyed, thus fewer replication sites are present than earlier in the syndrome.

HIV seems to be present in all components of human blood. Human blood is composed of red and white blood cells; platelets, which help in blood clotting and scab formation; and plasma, the fluid. People receiving blood transfusions have caught AIDS from both whole blood and blood components.

The concentration of HIV in the blood is high compared to other bodily fluids. However, when comparing the blood concentration of HIV to another well-known blood-borne virus, hepatitis B, the concentration of HIV is low. HIV averages 10^4/milliliter; HBV averages 10^{13}.

HIV and anti-HIV antibodies have been isolated from the same blood sample, indicating that the antibody fails to bind to the virus and is ineffective in stopping the virus.

Semen. Living HIV was isolated and cultured from the semen of AIDS patients. There appears to be a high concentration of viruses in the semen of HIV-infected males. Cell-free viruses were found in semen. It is not known whether the virus is present in pre-ejaculate fluid. Pre-ejaculate fluid oozes from the tip of the penis after prolonged sexual excitation, but before ejaculation.

Saliva. Live HIV has been isolated and cultured from the saliva of people with AIDS and ARC and from healthy HIV-infected individuals. The concentration of viruses appears to be very low in saliva in relation to that of blood and semen. Of the small number of infected people tested, reports are contradictory. In an early small experiment, HIV was extracted from 4 out of 10 ARC patients and 2 out of 6 healthy individuals. In another study, 3 out of 34 and in a third study, only 1 out of 81 saliva samples from HIV-infected people contained live virus cultures. To put some perspective on the findings, in the third study viruses were successfully cultured out of the blood of only half the AIDS and ARC patients in the study, so isolation procedures were not perfect.

Vaginal and Cervical Secretions. Living HIV has been isolated from the vaginal and cervical secretions of females. The *cervix*, located deep within the vagina, is the opening to the uterus, or womb.

The concentration of HIV in these secretions seems low. Also, the HIV isolated from these secretions was difficult to culture. Only one specimen was taken during sexual activity. The state of sexual arousal may be an important factor, since female secretions change character and increase in quantity during sexual excitement. Whether HIV is present in these secretions consistently is not known.

Tears. The concentration of HIV in tears is very small, and it seems to appear rarely in infected patients. In one study, only 1 of 7 AIDS patients were found to have HIV in their tears. Living HIV was isolated and grown from the tears of one AIDS patient. HIV has also been found to nest in the retina, found deep within the eye.

Mother's Milk. Living HIV has been isolated from mother's milk. In one case, it is suspected that a baby contracted AIDS from its mother this way.

Urine and Feces. Living HIV has been cultured from urine. No published studies have been performed on feces, although it is reasonable to assume that HIV can also be found in feces since HIV can infect cells in the rectum and large intestine. Also, there is growing evidence, discussed later, that exposure to feces can transmit AIDS.

HIV Survival Outside the Host

HIV is a fragile virus, not able to survive or remain infectious outside its host organism very long compared to another common, troublesome blood-borne virus — hepatitis B. Using extremely high concentrations of virus, concentrations not found in biological systems, researchers found that HIV could remain infectious for 3 days if dried and held at room temperature. However, even with these concentrations, a rapid decrease in infectivity was found in a matter of hours. In a water-based solution of human blood, HIV was able to survive at room temperature for 15 days, or 7 days at 37 degrees Centigrade (C).

Although HIV does not die seconds after leaving the body as commonly reported, these laboratory results do not suggest that HIV can be easily transmitted from the environment to a new host, or from human host to human host. All evidence indicates that HIV is rather difficult to catch. This information is more important to laboratory researchers than to the average human. HIV survival and methods of destroying it are discussed in Chapter 19.

HIV Transmission — Sexual

For a while, many researchers in the United States were skeptical about whether females could transmit HIV to males at all. There were no documented cases. Almost all HIV-infected people are male homosexuals, male hemophiliacs, and male IV drug users. The few HIV-infected females available for study have mostly been IV drug users and sexual partners of the aforementioned males.

Early in the AIDS epidemic, it became evident that females could catch AIDS from infected males. The wives of HIV-infected male hemophiliacs provided strong proof that males could transmit HIV to females through vaginal intercourse. However, it was difficult to find a proven case of a female transmitting an HIV infection to a male. For a long time, reports came from Africa and Haiti of bidirectional sexual transmission (both male-to-female and female-to-male), but nothing specific could be traced in the United States. In the United States, a small number of infected males denied any IV drug use or homosexual contact, but claimed frequent sexual encounters with female prostitutes. At that time a small number of prostitutes, mostly IV drug users, were infected, so those males might have contracted HIV infection from females.

Finally, a clear case was found. A female was infected by her husband, who engaged in homosexual activity during business trips. After her husband died, she became sexually involved with her male neighbor. He became HIV-infected. For a period of a year, they had engaged in vaginal intercourse accompanied by deep kissing. Unless other risk factors have been overlooked, this case demonstrates that HIV infection can be transmitted by traditional sexual practices.

It seems that HIV is not as transmissible as other sexually transmitted diseases (STDs); that is, in any one instance of sexual intercourse, HIV does not cause infection as readily as, say, gonorrhea or syphilis. Also, the little available information indicates that women are at a higher risk than men for contracting syphilis and gonorrhea. However, gonorrhea, syphilis, and most STDs display their symptoms soon after infection takes place. Therefore the patient generally gets treated and cured.

The situation is different with HIV, of course. No one knows how long the virus *incubates* (grows quietly without causing outward signs of infection) in its host. HIV's incubation period can last 2 to 5 years. The history of AIDS is still too young for the full story to be known. Very few HIV-infected people actually know the date they became infected. Consequently, infected individuals may be engaging in sexual activity with their partners for years before any warning signs develop. The greater number of sexual encounters, either with the same infected partner or with a number of different partners whose statuses are not known, the greater the risk of an infection.

There is one suspected case of a female transmitting HIV to another female. One female homosexual apparently transmitted an HIV infection to her female homosexual partner. The couple engaged in oral-genital, oral-anal, and digital-anal sex over a long period of time.

HIV transmission from an infected partner to an uninfected partner does not necessarily occur. Some uninfected people have had unprotected sex (no condoms) with infected partners over long periods of time and have not contracted an HIV infection.

Although the size of the AIDS epidemic is not fully known, it is possible that AIDS may not be widespread in the U.S. heterosexual population. Although AIDS may be widespread in the U.S. homosexual male population, this population is somewhat self-limiting: homosexual males are more likely to have sex with homosexual males than with heterosexual males or females. Being a heterosexual is no excuse for being sexually careless, however. The extent of HIV infections in heterosexuals in the United States is not known, but it is certain to exist. Many men and women have sexual intercourse with both men and women; many single and married men (and fewer women) have sexual intercourse with prostitutes.

The people who catch AIDS from sexual activity are not necessarily promiscuous (have sex with many people). There should be no mistake about it; it is possible to catch AIDS from only *one* sexual contact.

When AIDS first appeared, the media reported that the average homosexual male AIDS patient had 1100 sexual partners in his lifetime. This average was true for the first 50 male homosexual AIDS patients studied. These men, however, were exceptions in the homosexual population. They may have counterparts in the heterosexual population—men and women who devote their lives to sexual activity. Female prostitutes may easily exceed 1100 sexual encounters in their careers.

Whenever a doctor asks a patient about his or her sex life, the patient is not likely to provide full information. The same is true for patients asked about their use of legal or illegal drugs. Not all patients lie or bend the truth, but they are more likely to lie about sexual activity and drug use (frequently to themselves) than about other health-related activities. Unfortunately, doctors are strong father and authority figures, and patients often desire to please the doctor by giving traditionally acceptable answers. Therefore, any information concerning HIV transmission through sexual activity must be evaluated with this in mind.

Anal Intercourse. Anal intercourse involves inserting one person's penis, or some other object, into the anus of another person. Anal intercourse seems to be the most effective sexual way of contracting an HIV infection. The greatest risk of contracting HIV belongs to the receptive partner. The receptive partner is the person whose anus is penetrated. This is true, presumably, for homosexual or heterosexual anal intercourse.

Originally, it was thought that anal intercourse transmits HIV infection because the insertion of the penis or any other object into the anus often creates open bleeding wounds along the inside walls of the anus. These wounds provide a doorway for viruses in the insertive partner's semen to enter the receptive partner's bloodstream. This may occur. Now, however, it is believed that no damage to the walls of the anus is necessary, since HIV has been shown, *in vitro,* to directly infect cells in the rectum and colon. In addition, the direct infection of roving, immune-activated macrophages in the mucous membranes lining the anus also seems possible.

According to a statistical study, rectal douching after anal intercourse increases the risk of contracting HIV infection.

"Fisting" is the insertion of fingers, or the entire hand, into the anus. It might be considered a form of anal intercourse. According to a statistical study, the insertive partner in fisting has a risk of contracting HIV infection, but there is little statistical risk for the receptive partner. The insertive partner may be contracting HIV infection from contact with blood or feces. People's hands often have small, invisible wounds around the cuticles of the fingernails; these may provide doorways into the body for the virus. This increased risk for the insertive partner may be a statistical quirk. If the risk does exist, no one yet knows its true cause.

Figure 13: Relative Risks of Sexual Activities

Anal Intercourse: Anal intercourse carries the greatest risk of HIV transmission to the receptive partner. Presumably this is true for heterosexuals as well as homosexual males. For the insertive partner, a near statistical zero risk occurs. According to interviews with homosexual men, the estimated statistical risk of contracting HIV infection in unprotected (without condoms) anal interourse is 1 in 100. Of course, transmission could take place the first time, the hundredth time, or any time in between.

Vaginal Intercourse: According to interviews with heterosexual individuals, the risk of contracting HIV in unprotected intercourse is 1 in 1000.

Oral Sex: According to statistical studies among homosexual men, the risk of HIV transmission in oral sex is low. Oral-anal contact has a slight statistical risk of HIV transmission. The risk of oral-genital transmission is low and is not measurable in the populations studied. Stated in another way, the risk approaches zero, but is not zero.

Kissing With Exchange of Saliva: There is one suspected case of HIV transmission via kissing. The risk is low: 1 in some very large number. This risk seems close to zero, but is not zero.

Note: Interviewing is a very poor way to get facts. Individuals sometimes lie about their sexual activity, and subconscious distortion of facts is very common. The statistical risks here are unclear as the AIDS epidemic is still young.

Vaginal Intercourse. In vaginal intercourse, a man's penis, or another object, is inserted into a woman's vagina. HIV can be passed from males to females and from females to males, during vaginal intercourse. Vaginal intercourse does not seem to be as effective a method of transmitting HIV as anal intercourse. The mechanism of heterosexual HIV transmission is still unclear.

Apparently, HIV transmission from males to females occurs more effectively than from females to males. This seems true for most sexually transmitted diseases; the female is at greater risk. A male's exposure to the female is fleeting, but the male leaves potentially contaminated semen in the female. Usually the semen remains in the female long after intercourse is over. The longer a person is exposed to germs, the more likely he or she is to contract the disease.

Rectal douching seems to increase the risk of HIV infection in male homosexuals. Vaginal douching is generally believed to decrease a female's risk of contracting an STD, but this belief has little scientific support. More research is needed.

MALE TO FEMALE: If the male is infected, he deposits HIV-infected semen inside the female's vagina. The walls of the vagina are lined with mucous membranes. The virus may be able to enter the outer surface mucous membranes and reach the blood vessels inside. It is also possible that HIV directly infects the roving macrophages found in the mucous membranes. In addition, small bleeding wounds develop inside a woman's vagina for any number of reasons, and any wound, no matter how small, provides a doorway into the bloodstream.

Certain conditions can make a woman's vagina more susceptible to infection. For example, *cervicitis* (inflammation of the cervix) is a common condition in women, which makes the surface of the cervix and the vagina more likely to bleed. Cervicitis can be caused by IUD contraceptive devices and by sexually transmitted diseases such as gonorrhea, syphilis, and *Chlamydia* infection.

There is no current reason to believe that HIV infection needs a doorway into the bloodstream to infect the female through the vagina. Laboratory evidence indicates that HIV infection can take place in the absence of any vaginal or cervical wounds. Researchers infected a female chimpanzee by spreading cell-free, laboratory-grown HIV inside the chimpanzee's vagina, which is almost identical to the vagina of human females. The concentration of virus used was much higher than that found in natural sexual situations. The researchers thought they caused no damage to the vagina because there was no blood on the swab after spreading the virus. The researchers do not know whether the swab touched the cervix. The chimpanzee developed a condition similar to lymphadenopathy, an early symptom of HIV infection. This experiment suggests that HIV can penetrate the mucous membranes found in the vagina and establish infection.

Females probably do not have an increased risk for contracting AIDS during menstruation. Menstrual bleeding is actually the shedding of tissue lining the uterus (womb). Menstrual blood flows from the uterus, through the cervix, and into the vagina, and there is no wound for entry by virus-infected semen.

FEMALE TO MALE: Males can catch HIV infection from females, but the method of transmission is not clear. It may be possible for infection to come from contact with menstrual blood, which probably contains the virus if the female is infected, or from contact with a woman's vaginal and cervical secretions.

In males, the doorway for HIV may be a very small wound on the head of the penis, in the mucous membranes lining the urethra, or through glands found at the inside of the base of the penis. The condition of the cells lining the urethra may be important in male susceptibility to infection. The health of these cells may be affected by other STDs or other irritants.

Oral Sex. Oral sex is defined here as the contact of one person's mouth with the penis, vagina, or anus of another person. There are no proven cases of anyone contracting or transmitting HIV infection from oral sex, but, theoretically, such transmissions could occur. Infection could pass from one person's mouth to the partner's penis, vagina, or anus with saliva as the carrier.

The mouth is frequently exposed to germs; the hands constantly bring germs to the mouth. Thus the mouth is well prepared, immunologically, to repel invaders. Conflicting evidence exists on whether HIV can infect someone through the mouth's mucous membranes. Researchers were unable in two attempts to infect a chimpanzee by spreading the virus inside the animal's mouth. Like the chimpanzee-vagina experiment, the researchers used a swab and an extremely high concentration of viruses. However, a health care worker who had HIV-infected blood splash into her mouth became infected.

It is possible that the virus penetrates the mucous membranes of the mouth. In addition, any small wound in the mouth provides a doorway into the blood-stream for viruses in contaminated semen, vaginal and cervical secretions, or menstrual blood. Small wounds may include cold sores, bleeding gums (perhaps inflicted by a toothbrush or dental floss), and self-inflicted bites.

The most risky form of oral sex is mouth-and-penis sex, including male ejaculation. This activity brings semen with its high concentration of viruses directly to the mouth's mucous membranes. In one study of male homosexu-als who had AIDS, there was minor statistical evidence that swallowing semen increases the risk of HIV infection. Most scientists think, however, that HIV can-not survive in the stomach's acids. Most likely, HIV infection actually occurs in the mouth.

According to an early study of homosexual men, oral-anal contact ("rim-ming") carries a small increased statistical risk of transmitting AIDS. The infec-tive substance may be feces or blood.

Most AIDS studies are small. Most statistical studies have involved male homosexuals and have not established a link between oral sex and HIV trans-mission. With male homosexuals, the statistics say that anal intercourse is the one clear activity associated with HIV infection. It is possible that oral sex can transmit HIV, but so ineffectively that transmission cannot be measured with the small samples on hand. Transmission of HIV by oral sex among homosex-uals may be so rare that it is concealed by the effects of anal sex. In other words, virtually everyone who engaged in anal sex probably also engaged in oral sex. Oral sex may have had the effect of adding a single drop of water to a bucket—no one would notice the difference. Statistics are not real life and at this early stage of the AIDS epidemic, particular care is required in interpreting the facts.

Kissing. Kissing is probably not an effective way to transmit AIDS, but there is one case of possible HIV transmission through kissing. An elderly man con-tracted AIDS from blood transfusions during major heart surgery. His surgery left him impotent (unable to have intercourse). The man stated that his only sex-ual contact with his wife was deep kissing, which included the exchange of saliva. His wife became infected.

Another factor which must be considered when discussing kissing is the presence of blood in the mouth. If a person is infected, blood contains a high concentration of the virus and is far more infectious than saliva alone. The presence of blood in the mouth is a common event, originating from bites, abra-sions, and bleeding gums. Kissing, if done roughly, can also create bleeding points in the mucous membranes of the gums and cheeks.

Kissing is evidently an extremely ineffective way of transmitting HIV. First, saliva in infected people does not always contain the virus. On limited evidence, the occurrence of HIV in the saliva seems infrequent and when HIV is present it is present in low concentrations. Finally, saliva has germ-killing abilities which are somewhat effective against HIV. However, kissing is so common and fre-quent that it seems possible that a rare case or two of HIV infection could be transmitted this way if the carrier population becomes large enough.

Figure 14: Other Sexually Transmitted Diseases (STDs)

Quite often, when a person catches one STD, he or she has been exposed to several. Condoms are thought to reduce the risk of contracting most STDs. Exposure does not mean that one always catches the disease. Here are a few common STD's.

Chlamydia. Probably an unusual form of bacteria, Chlamydia is now thought to be the major cause of non-specific urethritis. Infection may be asymptomatic or accompanied by mild symptoms; more severe itching and inflammation can often be cured with drugs. Possible cause of pelvic inflammatory disease (PID) in females, perhaps leading to sterility.

Genital Warts. Caused by the DNA papillomavirus, genital warts receive far less attention than most other STDs. Genital warts are associated with certain cancers in the penis or vagina, though they may or may not be the causative agent of these cancers.

Gonorrhea. Caused by bacteria, the usual symptom is a sensation of burning on urination, usually more noticeable in males than females. Often the cause of pelvic inflammatory disease (PID) in females, it is serious and possible deadly if left untreated. Long-term infection can cause sterility.

Hepatitis B. Hepatitis is the inflammation of the liver. It can be caused by viruses, chemicals, and other things. Hepatitis B is caused by a DNA virus. Symptoms are fatigue, diarrhea, headache, joint pain, and jaundice; a yellowing of the skin and eyes. Hepatitis B, left untreated, can be fatal.

Herpes. Genital herpes is caused by the herpes simplex virus. Herpes infection may be asymptomatic, or have stages in which painful blister-like sores develop. Episodes of blistering may be related to general health, stress, or irritation of the infected area by friction. The initial episode is usually the most painful.

Syphilis. Caused by a spirochete, a sort of bacteria. *Primary syphilis* may be asymptomatic or may develop as painless, open blisters or sores called chancres. Chancres occur at the site of contact, usually on mouth, anus, penis, or vagina. Clearly visible on the male's penis, chances are often not visible in females because they form on the walls of the vagina or on the cervix.

Untreated syphilis can advance to its *secondary* stage, characterized by rashes, headaches, hair loss, joint pain, nausea, constipation, and fever. *Tertiary* syphilis may cause brain damage and insanity, joint destruction, heart damage, and blindness.

Many high-risk and infected individuals are being told that kissing is totally safe. This may not be wise. Until research clarifies this issue, avoid deep kissing (exchange of saliva) with large numbers of people. Also avoid exchanging saliva with anyone belonging to a high-risk group for AIDS, or, obviously, anyone showing the symptoms of AIDS or any illness.

Urination. Contact with urine of a sexual partner (sometimes termed "water sports") is not advised because HIV has been isolated in urine and may be transmitted through microscopic lesions in the skin.

Sex Toys. In theory, viruses and other germs can travel from one host to another by means of artificial objects. If any sex toy comes in contact with contaminated body substances, it should be sterilized or disinfected before being inserted into any other body. Cleaning processes are discussed in Chapter 19.

HIV Transmission — Health Care Settings

Blood Transfusions. HIV seems to be present in most of the components of human blood: red and white blood cells, platelets, which help in blood clotting and scab formation, and plasma. People receiving blood transfusions have caught AIDS from whole blood and from blood components, including platelets, red blood cells, plasma, and clotting factor concentrates manufactured for hemophiliacs. Neither pasteurized (heat-treated) albumin nor gamma-globulin, two blood proteins commonly isolated and transfused into ill patients, have been reported to transmit HIV.

In 1985, a blood-screening test became available to blood testing centers, enabling them to screen all blood donations for HIV. The test's existence had another unfortunate side effect: Individuals started donating blood in order to find out if they were HIV infected. Also, not all high-risk individuals stopped donating blood. IV drug abusers have a long history of donating their blood in exchange for money. Despite these problems, the annual number of transfusion-related AIDS cases and HIV infections should soon stop. However, the blood test is not perfect, so some contaminated blood will slip through, and catching HIV from a heterologous blood transfusion (blood from a person other than yourself) will remain an extremely remote possibility. For more information on the AIDS blood test, see Chapter 7.

Clotting Factors. Clotting factors are concentrated proteins important in blood clotting and scab formation. The bodies of hemophiliacs do not produce enough of these proteins, so hemophiliacs must supplement them with clotting factors removed from the blood of other people. Several types of clotting factor concentrates exist; most have been responsible for HIV transmission. See the section on hemophiliacs in Chapter 12 for more information.

Hemodialysis. In hemodialysis, a person's blood is cleaned of body waste products and debris by a machine because the kidneys no longer function well. In the United States, 80,000 people require hemodialysis. Hemodialysis patients frequently have a history of blood transfusions and thus are at high risk for HIV infection.

Hemodialyzers (the machine mentioned above) are large and very expensive. They are located in hospitals or hemodialysis centers where patients come to them for treatment; thus the machines are shared by many individuals. The machines are cleaned between patients, so one patient's blood does not mix with another's. Any tubes or needles inserted in the body are sterilized before reuse or thrown away. Occasionally major blood spills occur; equipment, floors, and sometimes people get blood splashed on them, either during the accident or in cleaning up afterward. Where there are blood spills, there is risk of HIV transmission.

These sorts of accidents have transmitted the hepatitis B virus (HBV) in hemodialysis settings. HBV is a tougher virus than HIV and survives much longer outside the human body. HBV seems to be more infectious than HIV in needlestick accidents, probably because HBV concentration in the blood is much higher than that of HIV. The medical consensus is that the same medical precautions used to prevent hepatitis B transmission in hemodialysis settings will successfully prevent HIV transmission.

Organ Transplants. Anyone infected with HIV or thought to be at a high risk of having HIV infection should not donate blood, organs, or tissues for use in humans. This educational message is being spread by the U.S. Public Health Service and the Red Cross, but occasionally an infected person slips past the screening process. With organ transplants, several organ recipients also received HIV along with their donated organ. The problem has been one of time. Fresh organs must be used immediately. There is little time to wait for a blood test to see if the donor, who is probably dead, was HIV-infected. New, faster blood tests may change this.

Thus far recipients of liver, kidney, and skin grafts have contracted HIV infections from their donor organs or tissues. Transplants of the lens of the eye are very common and may also run a small risk of HIV transmission, since HIV is known to live in tissues of the eye.

Artificial Insemination. *Artificial insemination* is the use of a medical instrument to deliver a male's sperm to a female's vagina and uterus. This process is generally performed when the male member of a heterosexual couple is not able to effectively generate sperm, or if a female wishes to have a baby but does not wish to have a sexual relationship with a male.

A number of women have been exposed to HIV by artificial insemination. Little follow-up information is available. Other sexually transmitted diseases reportedly have also been transmitted by artificial insemination, including gonorrhea and *Chlamydia*.

Infected Health Care Workers. On rare occasions, health care workers infected with diseases transmit them to their patients. Cases of hepatitis B transmission are documented. Usually the infections appear in clusters with one health care worker infecting several patients before the situation is discovered. In one well-known case, a hepatitis B-infected oral surgeon infected four patients. Researchers in England estimate that the risk of receiving hepatitis B in a surgical operation is 1 case per 1 million operations per year. The risk stems from the surgeon cutting himself or herself and bleeding into the patient. At least one practicing surgeon in the United States has died of AIDS. A survey of 400 of his patients revealed no HIV infections.

Issues of infected health care workers are discussed in Chapter 19.

HIV Transmission — Other Forms

Pregnancy. HIV can cross the placental blood barrier, a barrier formed by chemical action to protect the unborn baby from disease and chemical substances. A baby in the womb can thus become infected with HIV. Fetuses 15 weeks old have been found to be HIV-infected. Approximately 70 to 90 percent of childhood AIDS cases are babies born to mothers with AIDS, mothers belonging to high-risk groups, or mothers whose sexual partners are members of high-risk groups. Presently, most children who have AIDS were diagnosed before 1 year of age.

Any woman belonging to a high-risk group or who is having sex with a member of a high-risk group or who tests positively for the presence of anti-HIV antibodies should avoid becoming pregnant. Pregnant women in this situation are often informed about the local options concerning abortion and, in the best circumstances, are provided with adequate psychological counseling to aid in the decision-making process.

Even if a mother is infected, it is possible that her baby may be born without being infected. The chances that an infant born to an infected mother will be infected range from 65 to 91 percent. These figures are based on a small number of mothers and infants. There are a couple of cases in which babies were apparently born with "passively" acquired antibodies—antibodies transmitted from the mother. These antibodies fade away over time.

It is possible that some babies do not contract the virus in the womb, but from exposure to the mother's blood during birth, or from mother's milk. One small study suggests that natural birth with its risk of exposure to mother's blood may represent a higher risk than cesarean section, where the baby is removed through a surgical opening in the mother's abdomen. There is one instance in which an infant seems to have contracted AIDS from its mother's milk.

Insects. Insects are known to transmit both viral and bacterial diseases to humans and other mammals. Insects commonly implicated in transmitting disease are mosquitoes, lice, bedbugs, ticks, fleas, and spiders. Insects are known to transmit both viruses and bacteria from animal reservoirs to humans, and probably vice versa.

Insects can be either biological transmitters or mechanical transmitters of disease. In *biological transmitters,* the cells inside the insect, in the salivary glands or gut for example, become infected by the pathogen (disease-causing organism). The insect becomes a virus-generating factory, capable of transmitting the disease for the remainder of its life.

Mechanical transmitters transmit pathogens from one host to another with mouthparts contaminated by infected blood. Mechanical transmission takes place when an insect is interrupted while feeding on one host and completes its meal on a second.

In theory, a person could be exposed to a virus by (1) being bitten, (2) crushing infected insects, and (3) rubbing the germs contained in the insect's feces into wounds when scratching insect bites. Some insects inject saliva or vomit food into the host before feeding, inserting potentially infecting pathogens into the wound.

A researcher has recently proved insect transmission of hepatitis B. Scientists of many disciplines disputed whether insects had any role in the spread of hepatitis B in the Third World. A single scientist's findings will not end a debate. Hepatitis B is primarly transmitted by sexual activity, the sharing of intravenous needles, and blood transfusions. Although hepatitis B is common in the United States, no insect transmission is known to occur. However, if insect transmission does occur, then its effect cannot be measured epidemiologically, meaning it cannot be seen by observing the spread of the disease amongst human populations. Such transmission must be proved by direct observation either in the field or in the laboratory.

Researchers have shown that hepatitis B can survive for up to 30 days within bedbugs, and during this time, be excreted in the insects' feces. In one study, about 15 percent of the bedbugs fed infected blood retained the hepatitis B virus. One researcher fed mosquitoes and bedbugs HIV-infected blood. The bedbugs kept HIV alive for over an hour; the mosquitoes apparently did not. This experiment proves little. Each virus and each host has its own story. Further research is needed, although it may not happen soon.

A discussion of virally induced encephalitis may add perspective to the issue of insect transmission. In 1986, 115 cases of encephalitis were reported in the United States, most thought to be transmitted by mosquitoes. Several different viruses were involved. In the same year, an astronomical number of mosquito bites occurred. Do these 115 cases of disease represent 1 case in 1 million bites? In 10 million? More? Less? Whatever the statistical risk, it is very small. Also, these viruses have been isolated from a number of hosts and carriers, such as mosquitoes, arthropods, bats, birds, rodents, and horses. HIV only has one known host.

In Africa, the low incidence of AIDS among children is frequently taken as evidence that insect transmission does not occur. A few dissidents disagree, saying that childhood cases are not always linked to mothers having AIDS and also reporting lousy (lice) living situations of some AIDS patients. Fortunately, the concentration of HIV is very low in human blood, reducing its ability to be transmitted.

In summary, insect transmission of HIV remains a remote possibility. If such transmission does exist, it is not epidemiologically important. Probably Human Immunodeficiency Virus (HIV) would become extinct if it relied solely on insect transmission. However, on the individual level, an infected person who claims never to have engaged in the designated risky activities, nor to have engaged in illicit sex, must be given the benefit of the doubt: that insects or other unknown methods of HIV transmission exist.

Intravenous (IV) Needles and Syringes. Intravenous needles are used by doctors to give injections of drugs or vaccines. IV drug users use these medical needles to "shoot up" (to inject illegal drugs), such as heroin or cocaine, into their bodies.

Intravenous means "inserted into a vein." IV needles and syringes (the plastic container attached to the IV needle) are both transmitters of HIV. Needles in doctor's offices are destroyed immediately after use, so they do not fall into the hands of IV drug users, who in the past raided the trash barrels outside hospitals.

HIV has spread very rapidly among some groups of IV drug users due to their reuse and sharing of needles. HIV is transmitted in the small amount of blood that remains in the needle or syringe after use.

In addition, several health care workers have contracted HIV infection by accidently sticking themselves with a needle containing the blood of an AIDS patient.

Another population possibly at risk are individuals who "shoot" steroids as part of a body-building or athletic regimen. Steroids are restricted substances, meaning that they can only be obtained with a doctor's prescription. An underground market in steroids exists as does a parallel market for hypodermic syringes. Again, since they are difficult to obtain, body builders are likely to share needles.

Contact with Bodily Secretions and Feces. There are a couple of cases in which HIV may have been transmitted through contact with feces.

In one case reported by the Centers for Disease Control (CDC), a mother was infected by her child. The infant was very ill at birth with physical problems that required surgery. The infant contracted AIDS from a blood transfusion. The mother performed many health care tasks for the infant, including giving injections, handling the infant's feces, inserting rectal tubes daily, drawing blood, and handling indwelling catheters, surgical dressings, and feeding tubes. The mother usually did not wear protective gloves and often did not wash her hands immediately after handling the baby and its excretions. The mother does not recall any needlestick accidents, but she had prolonged contact with the infant's feces, blood, saliva, and nasal secretions.

In another case, a nursing home worker in England developed HIV infection. She had prolonged contact with the bodily secretions and excretions of a man who died and was later assumed to have AIDS. She recalled having small cuts on her hands and a chronic case of eczema, a skin condition causing dry, pimpled, or chapped skin.

Blood-Letting Instruments. Any instrument which penetrates the skin or exposes blood should be carefully sterilized before reuse or broken so no one else can use it and discarded in puncture-resistant plastic bottles with screw-on caps. This includes ritual circumcision knives, acupuncture needles, tattooing needles or any instrument used to make scars or homemade tattoos, ear-piercing needles and equipment, and electrolysis equipment. Even the safety pins used by doctors during normal checkups to test sensitivity of the skin nerves should be carefully thrown away so that no one else can get stuck with them.

Personal Hygiene Equipment. Shaving razors and toothbrushes, both of which may come into contact with blood, may possibly transmit HIV from one person to another. Infected people should sterilize razors before discarding them or dispose of them in puncture-resistant containers.

Biting. There have been at least two cases of individuals being bitten deeply by an HIV-infected person. In both cases, no HIV infection occurred. A very small risk exists since HIV can be present in the saliva. For more detailed discussion of HIV in the mouth, see the section on kissing above.

Spitting. In a couple of instances, arresting police officers have been spit upon by infected people. No documented cases of infection from these types of situations have been found; however, a very small risk exists although it is probably too small to be measured.

Swimming Pools. Human viruses, such as enterovirus, rotavirus, and parovirus, have been known to survive in polluted water. Humans shed viruses into the water via urine and feces. They also shed respiratory and genital viruses into the water. HIV is primarily blood-borne and brain-borne, but small amounts may be present in urine and in semen.

For viruses to survive in pools, the chlorine levels must be inadequate or the pool must be poorly maintained: poor circulation, overload of people, or inadequate filtration.

People with open cuts, fresh abrasions, or open skin lesions should avoid pools and hydrotherapy to prevent both catching and transmitting disease. Most public health agencies have rules prohibiting individuals with infectious diseases from using public pools.

Animals. Any experimental animal which has been injected with or exposed to HIV may carry the virus and be able to infect a human if some exchange or transfer of contaminated fluids takes place. Thus far, chimpanzees seem to be the only primate that becomes infected with HIV. Few experiments with other nonprimate animals are reported.

HIV Transmission — None Found

Casual Contact. There is a great fear of catching AIDS through casual social contact, such as shaking hands or being in the same room with an infected person, touching doorknobs, or sharing bathroom facilities. The fear is far greater than the risk. Much of this fear may really be fear of other things misplaced onto AIDS. The potential consequences of giving in to this fear are discussed later.

Knowledge about the chances of catching AIDS from social contact is not likely to come from direct experimentation. Rather, it is likely to come from studying the progress of the disease in our society and around the world. Six years into the epidemic, casual social contact is coming up clean.

To date there are no known cases of AIDS or HIV infection transmitted by casual social contact, not even among people living in the same household. A growing number of small studies have examined the housemates and families of hundreds of AIDS patients. No cases of nonsexual HIV transmission have been found, even in situations where people frequently hugged, kissed, and shared toothbrushes with an infected person, although sharing of toothbrushes is not recommended.

No medical or health care workers are known to have contracted HIV through casual social contact with HIV-infected patients.

While the risk of catching HIV infection in casual social contact seems to be very near zero, it seems possible to catch other infections from HIV-infected people. In certain populations of HIV-infected people, there is a high occurrence of tuberculosis. Any person with tuberculosis is capable of transmitting it to others.

Other opportunistic diseases listed in Figure 10, namely, cytomegalovirus, herpes viruses, and toxoplasmosis, are a threat to infants, small children, and possibly to pregnant women and their fetuses. The immune systems of infants and small children are not fully developed, which is why they are not allowed to visit sick friends in the hospital.

Immunoglobulins. *Immunoglobulins* are large proteins which act as antibodies. Immunoglobulins are transfused or injected into people to help them fight infections. Immunoglobulins can be separated from whole blood. They were thought at one time to transmit HIV. Very large volumes of blood are needed to extract small amounts of immunoglobulins. This means that the blood of many people must be pooled together; thus the patient who eventually receives the immunoglobulins may be exposed to the blood products of dozens of people.

It was found that patients given immunoglobulin injections were testing positive for the anti-HIV antibody (anti-envelope/gp 120). Time revealed that these patients were not injected with live HIV virus which caused antibody production. Rather, the immunoglobulin injections contained anti-HIV antibodies. This is called *passive transmission* of antibodies. Since no HIV antigen is present, no new antibodies develop and the injected anti-HIV antibodies gradually fade away.

The immunoglobulin story illustrates the role of luck. Most commercially prepared immunoglobulin is separated by an ethanol fractionation process. Ethanol is drinking, or grain, alcohol. Ethanol is not as efficient at killing the virus as previously thought. It is possible that the ethanol fractionation process does not kill the virus, but that the HIV virus ends up in a fraction which is thrown away and only the antibodies end up in the final product.

Hepatitis B Vaccine. Around the time the AIDS epidemic began, a large number of male homosexuals received hepatitis B vaccine. Some of these men were part of vaccine trials, tests to determine the effectiveness of the vaccine. Vaccines are substances which induce antibody production, in this case anti-hepatitis B antibodies, without causing actual infection.

Hepatitis B is similar to HIV in that it is transmitted by sexual contact, blood transfusions, and the sharing of intravenous needles. Hepatitis B is very common in some urban male homosexual populations. Many doctors recommend that homosexual males get vaccinated against it. Many health care and dental workers, who are constantly exposed to blood, also receive hepatitis B vaccinations.

The hepatitis vaccine contains some human serum. Serum is basically plasma, the fluid part of the blood. Reportedly, serum is purchased in the Third World for commercial use in the United States. It was suggested that male homosexuals in the United States were inoculated with hepatitis B vaccine samples which carried HIV from the serum of HIV-infected people. HIV vaccine samples tested in 1986 revealed no detectable presence of HIV nucleic acids, and vaccine recipients historically have not developed anti-HIV antibodies following vaccination. In addition, anti-viral inactivation steps taken in vaccine manufacture proved effective in inactivating HIV.

Eventually, time and analysis revealed that the male homosexuals who were injected with the hepatitis B vaccine were not necessarily the same male homosexuals coming down with AIDS. Also, virtually none of the health care workers who received the vaccine came down with AIDS.

Cofactors of Catching AIDS

The Human Immunodeficiency Virus (HIV) is generally accepted as the causative agent of AIDS, although there may be one or a number of cofactors which are necessary to trigger HIV into action. Also, it is possible that something stands behind HIV, which makes it possible for HIV to freely replicate and cause visible damage.

In the early stages of the AIDS epidemic, it seemed that only 2 or 3 percent of infected people would progress into AIDS. This strongly suggested that these 2 or 3 percent were exposed to some other factor that promoted or triggered HIV infection. Yet time has revealed that the percentage of infected people who progress to AIDS has been steadily increasing. The people who have been infected the longest are at the highest risk of developing this serious illness.

Still, theories about the cause of AIDS are still expanding, fed by the streams of knowledge coming from reseachers the world over. An expanding number of possible contributing factors are being examined and reexamined.

Any one of the following may or may not be cofactors in contracting HIV infection. Also, the cofactors at work in one person may differ from those operating in another person. Finally, cofactors may not be necessary for AIDS to develop in all cases.

Immunodeficiency / Immunosuppression. Both words mean the same thing: The immune system is not working well. HIV causes immunosuppression by destroying T4-cells, but immunosuppression can exist because of a number of other factors.

Early in the epidemic it seemed likely that anyone who became infected with HIV did so while immunosuppressed. It was suggested by some researchers that only immunosuppressed people could contract the virus. A number of things cause immunosuppression, such as blood transfusions, pregnancy, legal and illegal drugs, certain viruses, and other germs. Some researchers report that immunosuppression precedes the appearance of HIV antibodies in the blood. The presence of antibodies is thought to indicate that the virus is replicating. Now it seems that immunodeficiency is not needed for HIV infection. However, immunodeficiency may play some role in the progression of the disease after infection has occurred.

Immune Stimulation. Laboratory information suggests that HIV can only infect lymphocytes that are "immune-activated," which means they have been stimulated into action by some other antigen. In the laboratory, HIV only grows in lymphocytes stimulated by laboratory antigens, called mitogens. "Resting" lymphocytes are not easily infected by HIV.

If the laboratory condition is the same in a living being, then HIV infection is probably more likely among people who are constantly being exposed to antigens or diseases. Lifestyle variables can also affect immune system function. A number of people in high-risk groups for AIDS are commonly in and out of immune-activated states. See the discussion about differences in AIDS patients in Chapter 12.

Genetic Factors. Every person in the world is different and unique. The instructions for building each of us, written in a chemical alphabet in our DNA strands, are all different in small ways. Just as our genes determine the shape of our nose or face, genes also determine the shape of our lymphocytes. It is possible that these differences in the lymphocytic shape or structure make some people more susceptible than others to HIV infection.

Three genetically determined factors have been statistically related to HIV infection and progression to AIDS. The first is HLA DR5. This stands for human leukocyte antigen DR5. A leukocyte is a white blood cell. Lymphocytes are a subgroup of white blood cells. HLA DR5 is simply a molecule that sits on the surface of a cell. This molecule is really a flag with the word "friend" on it. The immune system does not attack anybody waving a friendly flag.

Different people have different HLA flags. In some early studies, about two-thirds of the AIDS patients had the HLA DR5 marker. HLA DR5 is strongly associated with Kaposi's sarcoma in AIDS patients. For some unknown reason, the HLA DR5 marker does not seem as common among AIDS patients now as it was in the beginning of the epidemic.

In a small study, a second HLA marker, HLA B35, has been associated with greater likelihood of disease progression.

The third genetic factor is a group of proteins called Gc. There are three Gc proteins: Gc 1f(ast), Gc 1s(low), and Gc 2. (These are, respectively, homozygous, heterozygous, and homozygous; typical Mendelian inheritance.)

In a reasonably sized study, AIDS patients were significantly more likely than healthy individuals to have homozygous Gc 1f genes. All AIDS patients in the study lacked the homozygous Gc 2 protein, which seemed to offer protection against infection. Many of the uninfected symptomless people in the study had the genes for Gc 2. Some of these seronegative people were the sexual partners of AIDS patients. Presumably, these individuals were exposed to the virus, but did not contract it.

The Gc proteins are associated with the membranes of cells. Each of the three Gc proteins are structurally different in small ways. HIV probably has the easiest time binding to or entering cells with the Gc 1 structure on its surface. The same is probably true for certain HLA molecules.

If this tendency exists, then a person having the genes for these structures is probably more susceptible to HIV infection, and more susceptible to disease progression since the virus should be able to spread from one host cell to another with greater ease.

Possibly, the factors mentioned here are not the actual factors creating differences between AIDS patients. Perhaps the genes which create Gc 1 or the genes that create HLA DR5 are not the genes responsible for these perceived differences. Possibly, these genes merely sit near other more important genes on the same chromosome. Genes on the same chromosome all get passed along together. It is possible that gene products which we know nothing about are the determining factors in susceptibility to HIV infection and subsequent disease progression.

Two subsequent studies by other researchers failed to demonstrate an association between Gc types and the development of AIDS.

Cofactors in Developing AIDS Disease

Immunosuppression, immune activation, and genetic factors may also contribute to the progression of HIV infection and the development of opportunistic infections and abnormal conditions related to AIDS.

Additional factors may also promote the progression of the disease or determine which symptoms appear in an HIV-infected person.

Viruses. Viruses other than HIV may bring about immune suppression or activation, promote or trigger HIV replication, or contribute to T-cell death.

In male homosexual AIDS patients, there is a strong relationship between AIDS and the presence of the following viruses: cytomegalovirus (CMV), Epstein-Barr virus (EBV), herpes simplex viruses 1 and 2 (HSV-I and HSV-II), and human T-cell leukemia viruses 1 and 2 (HTLV-I and HTLV-II). Some of these viruses also infect lymphocytes. Figure 10 lists the diseases caused by these viruses. Also, scientists have found hepatitis B viral DNA inside HIV-infected T-cells. This surprised them because no antibodies for the hepatitis B virus were found. So HBV may be added to the list of possible cofactors.

Viruses often shed a number of chemicals. Theoretically, the shedding of two or more viruses could combine to create poisonous chemicals, or chemicals that interfere with the life processes of the host cell. So T-cell death could result from some cell-killing event that happens after viral replication.

It is also possible that some proteins made by one virus act as the promotor or trigger for the replication of another virus. In a different version of the story, one virus causes the host cell to create a protein which promotes the replication of another virus.

The Unknown Virus. An unknown and as yet unnamed virus has been isolated from AIDS patients. Its size apparently varies from the same as HIV to twice that. It does not appear to be a retrovirus.

Nonopportunistic Infections. Several diseases which infect uninfected "normal" people are being found in HIV-infected people. However, in HIV-infected people, these nonopportunistic infections tend to be more severe.

Syphilis, a common sexually transmitted disease (STD) has been discovered in small studies in a high number of AIDS patients. The odd thing about syphilis in AIDS patients is that it is not detected by the usual laboratory tests. It is often discovered in the brain after the patient has died. The brain is one of the primary infection sites for syphilis. Syphilis is being examined as a cofactor in AIDS progression.

Other long-lasting diseases caused by amoebas and parasites common to the tropics are suspected of causing long-lasting immunosuppression, potentially contributing to the progression of HIV infection in certain homosexual male populations.

Poppers. *Poppers* are small capsules of amyl or butyl nitrites. When the capsules are broken open and the chemicals inhaled, the heart starts beating rapidly and blood rushes to the head, creating a "high." Amyl and butyl nitrites have a medical purpose. In people with weak hearts, they stimulate the heart to beat rapidly, if inhaled as the heart begins to fail.

Statistics suggest that popper use promotes the development of Kaposi's sarcoma. In homosexual males infected with HIV, the use of poppers is associated with the clinical appearance of Kaposi's sarcoma. Kaposi's sarcoma is not AIDS; it is only one of the possible opportunistic diseases that some AIDS patients develop.

Another possibility suggested is that the use of poppers is a marker for sexual promiscuity. Evidence is growing that Kaposi's sarcoma has a viral cause. Perhaps this virus is contracted during frequent sexual activity with many people.

Among male homosexual AIDS patients, almost 50 percent had Kaposi's sarcoma during their initial diagnosis. Among heterosexual male IV drug users, only 3.8 percent had this condition. Presumably, homosexual males are being exposed to some other factor which promotes the development of Kaposi's sarcoma.

Nutrition. In all long-lasting diseases in which a germ gradually breaks down its host, nutrition is an important factor in maintaining the host's health. AIDS patients are known to lose weight drastically.

Some of the opportunistic diseases in AIDS, such as Kaposi's sarcoma, damage parts of the gastrointestinal tract (stomach and intestines). As a result, nutrients cannot be absorbed from food.

Malnutrition also causes immunosuppression. So weight loss and malnutrition and efforts to fight these conditions may affect the progression of HIV infection and the appearance and development of opportunistic infections.

Mental and Emotional State. Mental attitude and emotional state may affect the course of disease. This issue is discussed in greater detail in Chapter 9.

Geography. The climate in which an AIDS patient lives also affects which opportunistic disease germs the patient is likely to encounter. In temperate regions, *Pneumocystis carinii* pneumonia (PCP) is more likely to develop. In the tropics, PCP is rare, but cryptosporidiosis, enteritis, toxoplasmosis, fungal infections, and tuberculosis are more likely to develop.

The Smallpox Vaccine. A disputed theory related to the origin of AIDS concerns the smallpox vaccine, widely distributed in massive campaigns to rid the world of smallpox. The smallpox vaccine contains the *vaccinia* virus, frequently used in genetic engineering and vaccines. The Vaccinia virus has been known to trigger other viruses into action.

The smallpox vaccine is suspected as a cofactor because it apparently triggered the rapid development of AIDS in a previously asymptomatic U.S. army recruit.

6. Detecting AIDS

The detection of HIV infection in its early stages remains a problem. The physical symptoms are vague, and often attributable to other common illnesses. Laboratory tests reveal HIV's footprints but have little prognostic value, meaning they hint that HIV is present but cannot predict disease progression. As outlined in the CDC surveillance definition, there are multiple pathways of detecting and defining HIV infection (AIDS).

Initial Symptoms

The initial symptoms of AIDS are the same as the symptoms of lymphadenopathy, namely, fever, night sweats and chills, weight loss, diarrhea, sore throat, swollen glands, difficulty in swallowing (dysphagia), fatigue, and depression. Some, all, or none of these symptoms may appear in an HIV-infected person. Obviously, many of these minor ailments may be temporarily caused by a number of other illnesses. In HIV infection, these symptoms may persist for months without apparent reason. In any persistent illness, a doctor should be consulted.

Acute Reaction

A number of people have an acute reaction to HIV infection. Acute means that the reaction begins and ends quickly. The symptoms are severe but usually last a short time.

Some researchers describe the acute reaction as being similar to the flu; others call it mononucleosis-like. Historically, the acute reaction appears 3 to 12 weeks after exposure, apparently coinciding with the appearance of antibodies in the blood. This reaction could be directly caused by the HIV, or be caused by the reactivation of some other virus (cytomegalovirus is suspected).

The symptoms of the acute illness are, generally, fever, tremors, joint discomfort, headache, temporary lymphadenopathy, and muscle aches. Less frequently observed are pimples or rash, abdominal cramps, diarrhea, and hives.

Oral and Facial Signs

The mouth, face, head, and neck are the areas where the first visible signs of HIV infection appear. In lymphadenopathy, the lymph nodes about the head, face, and neck are often the first to swell. They swell during other infections, such as a cold or flu.

In many ARC or AIDS patients, the mouth, face, and head are also where the first opportunistic infections occur. The most common are: (1) *oral candidiasis* (white spots or patches on the tongue or mucous membrane of the cheeks); (2) *oral hairy leukoplakia* (fuzzy white spots on the tongue caused by a rare mouth fungus which does not rub off in AIDS patients as the hairy tongue caused by smoking does); and, (3) *herpes zoster blisters* (large, painful, pus-filled pimples which follow the path of a nerve under the skin). Herpes zoster is not too uncommon in people who are not infected with HIV. See Figure 10 and Chapter 4 for more information on these opportunistic infections.

The appearance of any of these signs in a person at high risk for HIV infection should be a warning to seek a health evaluation.

Blood Tests

A person's blood can be tested for the presence of anti-HIV antibodies. Two tests are commonly used: the ELISA and the Western blot. The ELISA test detects the presence of anti-HIV antibodies in a person's blood. *ELISA* means enzyme-linked immunoabsorbent assay. Usually, the ELISA detects only the anti-envelope antibody (anti-gp120), directed against HIV's protein coat. If the ELISA tests find evidence of antibodies in the blood, then the individual is considered *seropositive.*

The ELISA test is very sensitive, meaning it detects small amounts of antibodies. However, because it is so *sensitive,* ELISA can be fooled by the presence of proteins or antibodies unrelated to HIV. A high percentage of ELISA seropositive results are false-positives. Consequently, in normal testing procedures, ELISA-positive samples are tested again. If the blood sample continues to test positive by ELISA, then testing by Western blot follows. The Western blot test is reserved as the confirmatory test because it is more difficult to perform, thus more expensive. Also, the Western blot test is not as sensitive as ELISA. Rather, the Western blot is very *specific,* meaning more exact in what it "sees." The specificity of the Western blot test eliminates most of ELISA's mistakes.

In the screening of potential blood donors performed by the American Red Cross, approximately 1 percent of all blood samples reacted positively on the first ELISA test. When these blood samples are retested by ELISA, approximately one-third are "repeatedly" reactive, representing approximately 0.35 percent of all the blood samples. With repeat testing, the ELISA is claimed to be 99 percent accurate. After Western blot testing, only 0.025 to 0.04 percent of all blood donors were both ELISA and Western blot positive for HIV.

If a person's blood tests positive using both tests, it is very likely that the individual's blood contains antibodies. If an individual has HIV-antibodies, then HIV is likely to be present, or was present in the past.

More Information on Testing

There are a number of ways to test for the presence of HIV in humans. Testing for the presence of anti-HIV antibodies (gp120) is the best method available for public screening thus far.

Research on better testing methods is continuing. Testing kits that give immediate results, that can be used in the home, or that detect anti-HIV antibodies in the saliva rather than in the blood are being developed. Soon, commercial tests will be available that directly detect HIV in the blood.

Antibody responses are usually strongest during lymphadenopathy syndrome. Researchers sometimes report difficulty in detecting antibodies in the advanced stages of HIV infection. The lack of antibodies may indicate (1) a decrease in HIV because it has killed off most of the patient's host cells and has nowhere to replicate, or (2) failure of B-cells which manufacture antibodies, or their triggering agents.

ELISA. To create the ELISA or other immunoassay kits, manufacturers first grow cultures of HIV, chemically "crush" the viruses, then spread the proteins of the virus coat (gp120) over the surface of beads (or inside tiny wells in a plate). Beads serve as artificial viruses so when a patient's blood is spread over a bead, any antibodies in the blood latch on to the bead. After a series of steps, dyes are spread over the bead to reveal the presence of any antibodies. If antibodies are present in the blood and they stick to the bead, then dye sticks also. If antibodies are not present then very little dye sticks. The amount of dye and the intensity of color remaining on the bead is proportionate to the number of antibodies present.

An expensive machine, a spectrophotometer, reads the intensity of color or, more accurately, it reads the *absorbance value*. Above a certain level of color (absorbance value) the person is considered *seropositive*. Below a certain absorbance value the person is *seronegative*. Usually, the absorbance value is set too low, sweeping some borderline cases into the seropositive arena, resulting in a high number of false-positives. The logic is that detecting a few false-positives is preferable to letting any false-negatives slip past.

Different manufacturers use different virus strains as their source culture. Thus different commercial products may vary in their ability to detect HIV strains. For example, the immunoassay kits used to test for HIV-1 in the United States are unable to detect HIV-2. In the future, crushed protein coats from many different strains will have to be included in each test kit.

There are a number of disadvantages to the use of the ELISA test. ELISA has a period of poor sensitivity—the "window" period. The *window period* is the time period between actual infection and the point where antibodies are detectable in the blood. During this time, for example, blood donors could be giving HIV-contaminated blood.

When ELISA was first made available some problems with test techniques were also reported, but manufacturer's instructions have dealt with these.

In addition, the HIV used in the ELISA test kits is grown in human cells. As a result, a few people test positive because their blood contains antibodies similar to the cell type in which HIV was grown.

Intravenous (IV) drug users seem to have high rates of both false-positives and false-negatives. IV drug users are known to have a high percentage of false results on other standard laboratory tests, possibly due to an excess of various antibodies, generated by all the antigens infecting their bodies. In sharing needles, IV drug users inject other people's blood cells and skin cells into themselves along with the drug. These foreign cells are antigenic invaders.

People who have had multiple blood transfusions may also have an excess of antibodies, which might induce a high percentage of false-positives.

Western Blot. The Western blot test is not a good general screening test for HIV. ELISA is more sensitive, better at picking a positive result out of a crowd. Western blot can then determine if this positive is really caused by HIV and not some other boogeyman; Western blot is very *specific*.

For the Western blot test, manufacturers crush cultured viruses and distribute their proteins into distinct "bands" on a gelatin paper using an electrical charge. While the ELISA kits only contain HIV's envelope protein (gp120) and detects only the corresponding anti-gp120 antibody, the Western blot test enables technicians to detect other anti-HIV antibodies by exposing the gelatin paper to blood. Antibodies in the blood latch onto the appropriate viral protein such as the transmembrane protein, core protein, or their precursors. In different people, the strength of antibody reactions differs—the bands on the paper differ in darkness. Some or all of the bands may be present. At this point technicians must interpret the results and, using their experience, determine whether the Western blot results confirm the ELISA test.

Antigen Test. Pending Food and Drug Administration approval is a blood test that directly detects the presence of the HIV envelope protein (antigen) in the blood. The antigen test has been available in Europe since 1986, where small studies indicate that the test may have some prognostic value. Whereas the other tests described here detect antibodies to HIV, the antigen test directly detects the presence of the gp120 protein in the blood.

In limited studies in Europe, antigen tests have been able to detect the presence of HIV as soon as 2 weeks after infection. The antigen test also provides a method of measuring the levels of HIV present in the blood, thus providing a method for directly measuring the efficacy of drugs.

In limited studies, researchers found that antigens appeared in the blood first—followed by antibodies. If the presence of antigens reemerged, then the patient was more likely to progress into ARC or AIDS.

How to Get Tested

If you suspect you are infected, or just wish to know your HIV status, DO NOT go to your local Red Cross clinic and donate blood in order to get tested. It is possible that a false-negative test result would place contaminated blood into the blood supply.

A few phone calls should locate a testing center near you. Individuals may, however, want to travel a distance to testing centers better suited to their needs. The Centers for Disease Control (CDC), a branch of the U.S. Public Health Service, has established a number of free test sites around the country. These offer an alternative to local doctors or hospitals, and guarantee confidentiality for the person being tested.

These alternative test sites are not evenly distributed around the country. They are located in areas where AIDS is most common. Sometimes alternative test sites are set up by community request. Free or inexpensive AIDS testing centers have also been set up by state governments and a number of other organizations.

Testing centers differ in quality, confidentiality, time it takes to get a test appointment (ranging from no appointment necessary to 2 months), and time it takes to get test results (2 days to 3 weeks). It may be wise to call and question the testing center about their procedures before arranging an appointment. Ideally, a person receives education and psychological counseling both before antibody testing and before receiving the results.

If a person tests negative, but belongs to a high-risk group or suspects exposure to HIV, then the tests are generally repeated at 3-month intervals for 6 months to 1 year.

Confidentiality

When something is kept confidential, it is kept secret. People who are seropositive may wish to keep their antibody status secret because many people have lost their jobs, their apartments, and their friends after their seropositive status became known. Also, seropositive people or even people at high risk for being HIV-infected, may not be able to get health insurance. Without health insurance, a person must be very rich to pay for the medical expenses of AIDS.

Tests performed by doctors and hospitals are not necessarily confidential. In some areas, doctors, medical-testing laboratories, and hospitals are required by law to report seropositive people to the local health authorities. In addition, any tests performed in these settings are recorded, either on paper or in a computer. Generally, these records can be obtained by a court-ordered subpoena.

Some physicians have tested their patients without telling them. Others have withheld test results from their patients. These sorts of abuses happened at larger hospitals in urban centers in the early years of the epidemic. Now, most large centers have rules to prevent these practices. However, these abuses are now being reported in hospitals in smaller urban and nonurban areas.

When a person enters a hospital he or she generally signs a consent form which allows the attending physician to order any diagnostic tests necessary. In some areas, new laws require doctors or hospitals to get informed consent from the patient before testing for HIV infection. *Informed consent* means the patient has been educated and understands the test's purpose, how the test works, the diagnostic potential of the test, and the consequences of the test.

The laws protecting the confidentiality of the patient vary from state to state. Your city or state health department or local AIDS service organization should have information on local laws.

Lists. At blood donation centers, it is current practice to keep lists of deferred donors, whose blood has been discarded. Deferred donors are people whose blood tested positive on the ELISA test; their blood may not have been repeatedly reactive or Western blot positive.

In some cases, a person's name is added to the list without his or her knowledge. It is common practice to allow the person to donate blood again, but the blood is simply discarded again. The confidentiality of these lists is in question.

What a Positive Blood Test Means

If a person's blood contains antibodies to HIV, this means one of three things.

First, the person was exposed to HIV, but his or her antibodies defeated the virus and the person no longer carries the virus, just the antibodies. There have been a handful of people, several men and at least one woman who tested positive for anti-HIV, but later tested negative. In a couple of instances, while

Figure 15: HIV Screening Programs

Immigrants.	People with certain infectious diseases are not allowed to immigrate to the United States. The U.S. Immigration Services keeps an official list of these diseases, and AIDS (HIV infection) is expected to be added to this list. In the future, immigration applicants or anyone applying for resident alien status can be required to take the AIDS test. In addition, legal alien residents who are seropositive could be deported.
Insurance.	Insurance companies wish to screen out seropositive applicants and/or people at high risk for becoming infected. As of fall 1987, very few states in the U.S. have forbidden insurance companies to test insurance applicants for HIV. In some states, AIDS test results are protected by law. In general, doctors are not legally obligated to report test results to insurance companies. However, this does not keep insurance companies from trying to get the information. In some areas, insurance companies have distributed, along with their traditional forms, standing requests for ELISA test results. The manner of distribution has made some doctors think that the AIDS test information is required for the insurance voucher to be processed.
International Travelers.	A number of countries world-wide are considering policies and procedures that would prevent any HIV-infected foreigner from entering their country. Reportedly, several countries already refuse visas to HIV-infected individuals.
Job Corps.	All volunteers are tested and seropositive individuals rejected.
Marriage Licenses.	AIDS testing as a requirement for marriage licenses is being considered by a number of states. Testing for other STDs such as gonorrhea and syphilis is a requirement for a marriage license in many states.
Military.	The U.S. Department of Defense screens all applicants seeking to join any branch of the armed services and also screens enlisted personnel. Applicants who test positive are rejected for military service. Seropositive servicemen are given restricted assignments.
Peace Corps.	All volunteers are tested and seropositive individuals rejected.
Red Cross.	The blood gathered by the Red Cross is used for medical operations or emergencies wherein people need to replace lost blood. The American Red Cross tests the blood of all people who donate blood.
State Department.	Currently, all current and prospective foreign service officers, and their children over the age of 12, must submit to testing. A seropositive employee is excluded from most overseas positions. If applicants or their family members test positive, they are rejected for service.

seropositive, the person had low T4-cell counts. Their T-cell counts improved with time. The immune systems of these people may have defeated the virus. It is also possible that the tests were wrong.

Second, the person is still carrying the HIV virus, but will not develop any AIDS-related illnesses.

Third, the person is carrying HIV and eventually will develop lymphadenopathy syndrome (LAS), AIDS-related complex (ARC), or AIDS. According to current information, about 36 percent of HIV-infected people will develop AIDS within 6 or 7 years of infection, with an additional 30 percent showing some clinical symptoms in that period.

In most animals, retrovirus infections last for the lifetime of the host. In humans, HIV infections have been shown to last for years. The AIDS epidemic is not old enough for us to know the end point of infection in the majority of cases. It now appears that an increasing percentage of seropositive people are slowly progressing toward clinical illness. The longer a person has been carrying the virus, the more statistically likely it is that he or she will get ill.

Accuracy

These blood tests are accurate but not perfect. Both false-positive and false-negative results can and do occur. In false-positive results, the test is fooled by proteins that look like the anti-HIV antibody. The ELISA test is recognized to be very accurate when used to test a high-risk population. However, in low-risk populations, a positive test result has a higher statistical likelihood of being a false-positive.

Another problem is that antibodies do not develop immediately. In limited instances, primarily involving individuals who had needlestick accidents, antibodies developed 3 to 12 weeks after infection. There are now indications that antibody development may require a year or more if HIV is contracted sexually. Also, some HIV-infected people do not develop anti-HIV antibodies or not enough to be detected in testing. HIV has been isolated and cultured from the blood of infected people having no clinical symptoms and no detectable antibodies.

Finally, different varieties of HIV exist. Different strains may have slight differences in their protein coats. Since antibodies are created to match the protein coat of a virus, anti-HIV antibodies differ from individual to individual and from HIV strain to HIV strain. Therefore, an ELISA test developed to detect one strain of HIV may not be able to detect another strain. This problem already exists. HIV-2, isolated in Europe and Africa, cannot be detected by ELISA tests for HIV-1, common to the United States, Europe, and Africa. This characteristic is viewed as a threat to the blood supply.

7. Treating AIDS

No cure for HIV infection exists. Yet notable advances have been made in treatment of both HIV infection and the opportunistic infections common to AIDS. These recent advances may significantly change the health and life expectancy of people currently infected; coming years will tell.

Most AIDS patients are treated by a team of doctors and therapists. Within the team, each specialist focuses on different aspects of HIV infection. The medical understanding of HIV infection is still growing. The future may bring the development of treatment strategies that individually address specific subgroups of HIV infection.

Experience has convinced many researchers that no single cure will soon be found. Rather, hope lies in *combination therapy,* consisting of a variety of drugs and substances to fight HIV infection directly, tackle opportunistic infections, and repair the damage done by both.

An overview of treatment approaches is given here.

Drugs

In many instances, drugs offer life and health. They do so at a price. Sometimes the price is small; sometimes the price is very demanding.

Most drugs are poisons (toxins). The best drugs are very poisonous to the germ, but only a little bit poisonous to the patient's body. In other words, the best drugs interfere with one or more life processes of the germ but do not adversely affect the patient's metabolism.

Most drugs have *side effects* – effects not wanted. Side effects may not be visible for a long time, but are almost always present. With a good drug, the germ is killed or some physical wrong righted, before irreparable damage is done to the patient by either the drug or the germ.

Dosage, the amount of drug given, is very important. Some drugs are not poisonous to the patient if given in small amounts. Our bodies can destroy and eliminate many toxins, if taken in small quantities. With some drugs, the poisonous dose and the therapeutic dose are very similar. Just a little too much medicine can kill. With an ideal drug, the therapeutic dose is very small, the poisonous dose is very large, and side effects give warning before the lethal dosage is reached.

After taking a drug for a long time, the patient or the germ may develop a *tolerance* to the drug, that is, the drug has less effect. Sometimes a higher dosage of the drug is required to achieve the same effect.

When fighting an infection with drugs, treatment should continue until all the germs invading the patient are destroyed. Stopping too soon may be harmful because only the weakest, most drug-susceptible germs have been destroyed, while the most drug-resistant germs have survived. These drug-resistant germs then reproduce, and a population of drug-resistant germs grows.

When two or more drugs are taken together, they may interfere with one another or they may increase the effects of each drug. For example, two antiviral drugs, AZT and ribavirin, when taken together, seem to cancel each other out. When a prescription drug is taken, no other legal or illegal drugs should be taken without the knowledge of the attending doctor.

Research and Development. Drug testing is a painstakingly slow process. It begins in the laboratory, testing the effects of drugs on germ cultures, and if experiments prove successful, the drug is then tested on animals. Humans follow animals in the testing process. After controlled human studies, the drug may be approved by the Food and Drug Administration (FDA) for public distribution, either as an over-the-counter or prescription drug.

In a *controlled human experiment,* one group is given the drug while a second group is given a fake drug. The two groups are statistically compared to see if the drug made the desired change in the first group. Sometimes these studies show that the drug has no curative effect. If both groups were composed of sick people and half the people in each group got well during the study, then these people probably got well on their own and the drug made no statistical difference.

This testing process normally takes years. In addition, hundreds of thousands of dollars can be spent in experimentation and subsequent FDA application processes. Usually, these costs are borne by drug manufacturers who are gambling that the money will return in drug sales. In some instances, drug experimentation is directed and supported by various government agencies and performed by various universities and specialized research organizations.

Preceding drug testing is drug selection. Which drugs will be tested? Most likely, the drugs chosen have the greatest potential for profit or the drugs are specifically identified by government agencies for government-funded research.

The Drug Underground. Dissatisfied with the progress of government and pharmaceutical drug research, a number of HIV-infected individuals are experimenting with drugs not approved by the FDA. Some of these drugs are legal in other countries and are smuggled into the United States. Other drugs are manufactured in homemade laboratories.

While there are probably substances that fight HIV better than AZT, no one really knows a drug's true effect until it is tested by scientific methods in controlled experiments or until large numbers of people have tried it over long periods of time. For example, ribavirin is suggested as a better option than AZT. Yet without large, controlled experiments, it is difficult to measure ribavirin's true effects. If a doctor gives a drug to 10 patients and 8 of them get well, this is not proof that these patients did not get well on their own. Or that this group, by a statistical fluke, could be the only group that will get well. Without direct comparison of large numbers of people in controlled situations, it is very difficult to measure the effects of a drug.

Another problem with uncontrolled studies is the "placebo effect." A person's health or perception of health can be affected by attitude. A person's health may actually improve with a sugar pill if he or she thinks the sugar pill will cure. And doctors can sometimes see what they want to see, convincing themselves

Figure 16: Experimental Drug Information

American Fund for AIDS Research (AmFAR). Largest AIDS-related non-profit research group, conducts laboratory and clinical studies. Publishes newsletter "AMFAR Directory of Experimental Treatments for AIDS & ARC." Subscription is $50; $69 Overseas. U.S. dollars only. Send checks to: Book Order Dept, Mary Ann Liebert, Inc., 1651 Third Avenue, New York, NY, 10128, or call: (800) 526-5368

AIDS Treatment News. Published biweekly by John S. James. Reports on experimental and alternative treatments. Gathers information from medical journals and interviews with scientists, physicians, and people with HIV infection. Subscription: $25 dollars per quarter year ($8 dollars for persons with AIDS or ARC); subscription includes important back issues. Send checks to: John S. James, P.O Box 411256, San Francisco, CA, 94141. (415) 282-0110

Project Inform. Distributes information on treatments not approved by FDA. Conducts research surveys of experimental drug users. Information packets available. Toll-free hotline: (800) 822-7422. In California (800) 334-7422.

---

that improvements are occurring.

In an attempt to overcome the lack of research on different drugs, several organizations are building a pool of knowledge, collected by telephone interviews and questionnaires, about patient experiences with various drugs. These organizations also distribute information on how to manufacture drugs or how to obtain them. Other organizations apply political pressure to speed up government research and to push certain drugs into the Food and Drug Administration (FDA) approval process. (See Figure 17.)

Although the FDA has streamlined its regulations, making it easier for dying patients to obtain experimental drugs, the FDA and other branches of the government are the targets of much criticism.

Many HIV-infected people need to express anger at some point during the course of their infection. The patient's loved ones often share this anger. This anger can have both irrational and rational aspects to it. Frequently, a substantial portion of this anger is directed at the government.

While the U.S. government is a world leader in funding AIDS research, much of this research is focused on the development of a vaccine, not necessarily directed at the development of effective treatment. And in the area of AIDS education, the United States is lagging behind all other Western nations.

AIDS is a hot political issue. No doubt, AIDS research and related drug research are subject to a variety of internal and external political forces. At some point, political expediency, not scientific knowledge, will likely determine research goals and the development of subsequent treatment options. Individuals and organizations can make a difference in this process.

Fighting Opportunistic Diseases

Death in AIDS patients is caused primarily by the diseases listed in Figure 10 and the associated conditions listed in Figure 11, and is not due directly to HIV infection. Deaths due directly to HIV infection probably involve brain damage. Since HIV infection, the cause of the immune system failure, cannot yet be cured, some members of the medical team focus on stopping or slowing the progress of the opportunistic diseases.

Doctors treat these illnesses with a variety of drugs. Some illnesses respond to treatment, only to recur after treatment stops. Some diseases do not respond to treatment. Experimental drugs are continually being tried, with varying success.

As a rule, drugs which have an immunosuppressive effect, blocking the action of the immune system, are being avoided. In the future, the suppression of the immune response may be attempted purposefully. Blocking the immune response could prevent HIV replication, if HIV actually relies on host cell activation (T4-cells, macrophages, B-cells) to trigger replication, as currently suspected. Future experimental drug treatments may encourage certain immune cells to remain inactive during germ invasion, leaving non-HIV invading germs to be destroyed by artificial chemicals provided by doctors.

Fighting HIV Infection

If the Human Immunodeficiency Virus (HIV) is the cause of immune system failure, then the virus must be destroyed or stopped. Destroying viruses is a difficult task. First, any viruses found in the blood must be destroyed. Then any HIV-infected cells, such as T-cells, B-cells, and macrophages, must be destroyed. Since HIV can directly infect some brain tissues, successful removal of HIV from the human body means some brain cells must be destroyed too. In addition, most drugs do not destroy the virus without damaging the host as well. Destruction presents so many problems that researchers are focusing on using drugs to stop viral replication, instead. Figure 17 outlines the approaches to stopping viral replication. Drugs developed to stop replication may be most effective in patients in the early stages of HIV infection before a large number of T-cells are destroyed.

Currently, worldwide, hundreds of drugs are being tested for their effectiveness in destroying HIV or stopping HIV replication. Information on the following drugs is provided here because of their proven efficiency, or because of the media attention they have received.

AZT (Azidothymidine). In Fall 1987 AZT was considered the best drug available, according to normal scientific standards.

AZT does not kill the virus; it stops viral replication. AZT apparently does this by fooling reverse-transcriptase, the viral enzyme that reverse-transcribes the RNA into DNA. Quite simply, reverse-transcriptase grabs AZT to use in building a chain of viral DNA. AZT looks just like the real building-block normally used, but AZT stops chain construction cold. Any link in a chain holds on to two other links. AZT is able to form only one link. Wherever AZT appears in a DNA strand, the strand ends there. Think of a chain of people holding

Figure 17: Targets for Drugs

Step	Stage	Intervention
1	Virus binding to cell	Stimulate antibody production. Develop monoclonal antibodies to block virus's epitopes (key) or, conversely, to block the receptor site (lock) on host cell.
2	Injection of RNA into cell	Develop compounds that block injection of RNA or reverse transcriptase into the host cell.
3	Reverse transcription of viral RNA into viral DNA, performed by reverse-transcriptase (RT).	If RT does not function, then the viral RNA is degraded by the enzymes of the host. Because RT is unique to retroviruses, disruption of RT activity should not directly affect human cell function. Thus RT is an excellent target for drug treatment and a major focus of research activity. Drugs which interfere with RT are AZT, Acyclovir, Suramin, and Ribavirin.
4	Viral DNA splicing into host DNA.	Perhaps block the activity of HIV's *pol* gene.
5	Transcription: viral DNA written to viral RNA replicas.	Use "anti-sense" chemicals that fool the enzymes into using artificial, useless building blocks where the real nucleotides should be used, something like using nonsensical words in a sentence.
6	Viral assembly	Block HIV's *tat* and *art* genes or disrupt their products. These gene products are necessary for reproduction at these stages. Or use "anti-sense" artificial building blocks.
7	Budding	Enzyme inhibition suggested. Alpha-interferon is thought to inhibit replication at this step.

Chemicals which prevent viral function before or during Step 3 prevent the virus from successfully infecting new cells. Drugs that affect the virus after Step 3 prevent viral replication within cells. Successful treatment of HIV infection might require the use of more than one type of drug.

hands; this chain ends at the person with one hand tied behind his or her back. In this way AZT prevents viral replication by preventing the completion of viral DNA strands.

AZT does not destroy any viruses that are not in the process of replication. If a patient stops taking AZT, the replication process starts again. An HIV-infected person must take AZT for the remainder of his or her life, or until some better treatment is found.

The advantages of AZT are: (1) it can be swallowed; (2) it is easily absorbed into the bloodstream from the stomach; (3) it is able to penetrate the blood-brain-barrier, which protects the brain and cerebral spinal fluid from foreign substances; and (4) it seems to alleviate the symptoms of both HIV infection and many of the opportunistic infections. In mice, AZT has been shown to cross the placental blood-barrier, which protects the baby in the womb. Thus in the future AZT may offer some protection to pregnant HIV-infected women.

Many patients treated with AZT respond to therapy by the second week, a quick clinical reponse. Many patients treated with AZT report they feel better, have more energy and less fatigue, have better appetites, and they experience weight gains. These patients, as a group, also have fewer bouts of infection, and central nervous system symptoms such as cognition, coordination, and peripheral nerve function improve. Some immune system changes also occur. The T4-cell count doubles or triples in some patients, and in some patients the ability to have a skin allergic reaction returns.

The disadvantages of AZT are its side effects. Some people experience headaches, nausea, or reductions of red and white blood cells. Most patients thus affected are able to tolerate a lower dose of the drug. Problems arise because AZT is toxic to the bone marrow, which manufactures blood cells. Patients may require multiple blood transfusions in order to keep their red and white blood cell counts up.

AZT has been tested on only a limited population of HIV-infected people, namely, those with ARC or people recently recovered from *Pneumocystis carinii* pneumonia (PCP). They must not have undergone any previous chemotherapy or have taken any drugs that affect bone marrow. This population was selected for initial testing by the researchers designing the initial drug trials. Currently, a large study is under way testing the effect of AZT in an asymptomatic population.

By Fall 1987 some HIV-infected people had been taking AZT for 2 years. This group experienced a significant reduction in death rates compared with untreated HIV-infected people.

The annual cost of AZT treatment is estimated at $8,000–$12,000. For patients fortunate enough to be properly insured, the personal cost may be reduced to several hundred dollars.

Very recently, Burroughs-Wellcome, the manufacturer of AZT, established a new distribution system for this drug. Initially, AZT was available only to physicians who enrolled in a program specified by Burroughs-Wellcome, who were participating in controlled drug trials. AZT is now available as a regular prescription drug. Any physician can prescribe it. Burroughs-Wellcome, located in Research Triangle Park, North Carolina, has a hotline for AZT information: (800) 843-9388. The service is primarily for the benefit of physicians.

Ribavirin. Ribavirin was one of the first hopes for an effective anti-HIV agent. It is relatively nontoxic and can be taken orally. Data is contradictory on whether it effectively crosses the blood-brain-barrier. The general consensus is that it does not. In early experiments, ribavirin seemed promising but researchers are having difficulty reproducing the beneficial results.

Ribavirin has not been approved for use in the United States for HIV treatment, but is available in some foreign countries, including Mexico. Some HIV-infected people are smuggling ribavirin into the United States. Ribavirin and AZT combined have been shown to cancel each other out in one study.

T8-cells. T8-cells suppress (block) the activity of T4-cells. For certain parts of the immune system, T4-cells are the gas pedal and T8-cells are the brake.

It has been shown, *in vitro*, that T8-cells inhibit HIV replication in blood cells. T8-cells release a number of communication chemicals, so it is possible that one of these chemicals directly suppresses HIV replication. It is also possible that the T8-cells suppress any activity of T4-cells, thus preventing triggering of HIV replication. The beneficial effects of T8-cells do not seem to stem from cell-killing activity.

The greatest experimental effect was found when the blood and T8-cells were both from the same person. The more T8-cells added, the larger the effect on the culture. These results open the possibility that T8-cells can be stimulated in humans or that T8-cells could be collected from donors and transfused into patients. These two techniques are still only theory.

Cytotoxic Cells. Cytotoxic cells are cells which kill other cells through a process called *lysis.* In lysis, cells burst open. Cytotoxic lymphocytes will attach to virus-infected cells and, using chemicals, cause the membranes of the infected cells to burst open.

In one experiment, a group of French and Zairian researchers inoculated themselves with a substance of vaccine potential, which reportedly stimulated their immune system to produce large numbers of cells able to kill HIV-infected cells. The researchers did not then "challenge" their immune systems with HIV, so the substance has not been proved effective. If the substance is effective, it may have potential for people already infected with HIV, in addition to having vaccine potential.

Monoclonal Antibodies. Monoclonal antibodies are laboratory-created antibodies. They are created by fusing a cancer cell and a human antibody-making B-cell. These cancer cells have the strange trait of immortality, meaning they live in the lab for long periods of time. The hybrid made of the cancer cell and the B-cell continually manufactures human antibodies. These antibodies can then be injected into humans to fight infections.

In theory, it should be possible to make HIV-specific antibodies that are able to neutralize the antigen and to draw killing cells to the site of infection.

Viral Interference. Retroviruses with similar protein coats are sometimes known to interfere with each other in the same host. This is called viral interference.

This phenomenon leads some scientists to think that a nondeadly form of HIV can be created in the laboratory and then injected into an HIV-infected person. For example, a safe HIV could be created that would quickly bind to T-cells and prevent HIV from attaching to these sites.

Other scientists warn against using any form of HIV. In some small studies, the HIV protein coat by itself destroyed some T4-cells, proving the danger of even parts of the virus. Also, there is no guarantee that a safe virus will remain safe after recombining its genetic material with the genetic material of its host or other viruses. In addition, the viral interference strategy will only work if the stem cells, created in bone marrow, are not infected.

Peptide T. Peptides are a special group of chemical compounds found in the body. They are generally subunits of larger molecules and are themselves made of subunits called amino acids. Peptide T has three units of the amino acid threonine, thus its name "T." Peptide T is artificially produced.

Peptide T looks like the protein molecules found on HIV's protein coat. Thus, it latches onto the receptor sites on T4-cells just as HIV does. But if peptide T gets there first, HIV is unable to find a binding site.

In vitro, peptide T blocks the infection of human cells by HIV. Because it resembles a peptide found in the intestines, peptide T is presumed to be non-toxic. Only small amounts seem to be needed to achieve the desired effect.

Four male homosexuals near death in Sweden were given peptide T. The treatment seemed to improve their health, but did not save their lives. Other experimenters have not been able to reproduce these results. Further studies are anticipated.

AL 721. AL 721 is a substance made from egg yolks. Researchers in Israel developed AL 721 while looking for a way to alter the function of receptor sites in cells. They later discovered that AL 721 affects protein coats of certain viruses. More exactly, AL 721 affects the lipid (fat or oil) composition of membranes. These changes in the composition of the virus adversely affect its ability to infect host cells. Viruses whose envelopes contain lipids include HIV, herpes viruses, cytomegalovirus (CMV), and the Epstein-Barr virus (EBV).

In vitro, AL 721 has been shown to reduce infection. It also had some positive results in two experiments involving some twenty-odd people, which is too few to prove anything. However, once these patients were taken off AL 721 treatment, their HIV infection progressed very rapidly.

AL 721 is made in other countries, but is not legally available in the United States. AL 721 substitutes are currently being made in bathtub laboratories in the United States. AL 721 is in a gray legal area because, by some definitions, it qualifies as a food not a drug, since it is extracted from eggs. After demonstrations, including instances of civil disobedience, drew public attention to the matter, the FDA announced that AL 721 will receive initial testing.

Balancing the Immune System

Various substances of both natural and artificial origin are being used in attempts to control the function of the immune system. These substances are sometimes called *immune modulators* or *immunomodulators*. In this book, they have been referred to as communication chemicals. They are produced and released by cells of the immune system, either in response to some antigen or in response to some other signal of the body or immune system. The human body produces a vast array of these chemicals.

Interferons. Interferons are proteins, naturally produced by cells infected with viruses, which prevent viral replication. The interferons used in HIV therapy are made by genetically engineered bacteria into which enzyme-making genes from other organisms have been inserted.

Alpha-interferons are produced by white blood cells in response to viral antigens. In treatment, they have been found effective against HIV-related Kaposi's sarcoma and also against hairy cell leukoplakia. The best response is noted in patients without systemic (whole body) problems or previous opportunistic infections. These patients are thought to have a greater degree of intact T-cell function. Alpha-interferon's side effects include a flu-like syndrome with fever, headache, and nausea, with mild toxicity to bone marrow.

Gamma-interferon is produced by lymphocytes in response to antigens and affects antibody production and cell-mediated immunity through antibody-directed cell-lysis. It seems beneficial in some HIV-infected people.

Transfer Factor. No one is exactly sure what transfer factor is, but it appears to transfer immunity to infectious disease from one person to another.

Using pooled transfer factor from many people, researchers were able to improve the immune response, measured by lymphocyte proliferation and better skin reactivity, of some HIV-infected people. The improvements diminished after treatment stopped.

Interleukin-2 (IL-2). Interleukin-2 is a chemical produced by T-cells which triggers the immune response. T-cells infected with HIV do not seem to produce or release this chemical as they should.

IL-2 is also known as T-cell growth factor. It stimulates T-cell proliferation and regulates the function of T4-cells, T8-cells, and killer cells. The size, duration, and specificity of the T-cell functions are greatly influenced by IL-2. It may affect B-cells directly by changing the rate of B-cell proliferation, and indirectly because T-cells trigger B-cells.

IL-2 has been shown, *in vitro,* to increase skin reactivity, macrophage activity, lymphocyte proliferation, and gamma-interferon production by T-cells. It also increases natural killer cell activity and cytomegalovirus cytotoxic activity in both the laboratory and in humans.

Reconstructing the Immune System

Even if HIV were destroyed and the opportunistic diseases defeated, the patient would not remain healthy unless the immune system was repaired. The missing components must be temporarily replaced until the body can replenish them on its own. The following are strategies for replacing these components.

Lymphocyte Transfers. Lymphocyte transfers are transfers of white blood cells. Collections of white blood cells from healthy patients are injected into an HIV-infected patient's veins.

Bone Marrow Transplants. Bone marrow, a tissue found in the hollow centers of bones, manufactures white blood cells. Bone marrow seems to harbor or be infected by HIV, probably carried there by macrophages. Infected bone marrow may directly infect new white blood cells as they are created.

It is probably for this reason that bone marrow transplants have had little success in HIV-infected people. The transplanted marrow becomes reinfected. Also, the transplant patient is severely immunocompromised, due both to bone marrow trauma and to immunosuppressive drugs used to keep the transplanted bone marrow from attacking the body of the transplant patient. Bone marrow transplants do not yet represent any major treatment hope.

Thymic Transplantations. The thymus houses T-cells while they mature. It may also be a source for infection of new cells. Thymic destruction is suspected in many HIV-infected people and is very evident in children. The thymus has been mentioned as another possible site of immune reconstruction. These concepts are still in the theory stage.

Fighting Weight Loss

In many chronic diseases which can lead to death, the patient's nutritional status greatly affects the length of survival. The body's energy reserve may determine the time of death as much as the effects of the disease itself. Also, malnutrition adversely affects immune system function.

In and out of the hospital, caregivers are being instructed to make greater efforts to encourage and entice patients into eating, despite loss of appetite. In the hospital, the importance of artificial methods of feeding patients, once they are not able to feed themselves, is being reexamined. Patients can be fed nutrients through the veins or directly to the intestine, usually with a tube that goes up the nose, down the throat, and into the stomach. However, these practices increase the risk of infection or other complications in the weakened patients. Also, these are treatments patients might choose not to receive.

Alternative Health Care

The term *alternative therapies* refers to a group of health treatments or practices, some based on old traditions of various cultures around the world. Without doubt, some of these therapies and practices are beneficial to the practicing individual when properly applied. Unfortunately, these therapeutic techniques have all but been ignored by the scientific and medical establishments. A minority of individual physicians promote and apply various holistic principles and practices. However, there has been an appalling lack of controlled study involving holistic or alternative therapies.

This situation will undoubtedly change, just as the view of the importance of diet in relation to health has changed. Even as recently as 1960, the majority of doctors did not accept the concept that diet was the cause of a number of cancers and other ills. Yet, in the past 2 decades, research has demonstrated those strong links.

When holistic techniques undergo controlled studies, some demonstrated positive effects will likely be developed into more precise health tools. Others will prove to have lost their potency in environments or cultures that no longer resemble the circumstances of their origins.

Most likely, some holistic practices are beneficial. Holistic practices enhance overall health, and they do not have the drastic and costly effects of targeted drug treatments. Yet HIV infection is a war of attrition. Slowly the syndrome progresses, slowly the patient's defenses crumble. Perhaps some proportion of patients will benefit from holistic therapies.

A few alternative therapies currently being tried with AIDS patients are: (1) stress reduction, including: meditation; biofeedback; visualization of pleasing or healing images in one's mind; affirmations by thinking or reading positive, purposeful statements; hypnosis; and life planning; (2) macrobiotics, a discipline of eating based on certain principles of physical, emotional, and psychic balance; (3) acupuncture; (4) massage; and (5) chiropractic approaches.

For more on alternative therapies, contact a local AIDS organization or the Alternative Therapies Subcommittee, AIDS Action Committee, 661 Boylston Street, Boston, MA 02116. (617) 536-7733.

8. The Psychosocial Aspects of AIDS

Reactions to Diagnosis

When AIDS is diagnosed, patients confront more than possible death. HIV-infected individuals may face abandonment by their sexual partners, friends, and family; loss of their jobs through discrimination or incapacity to work; loss of their apartments through discrimination or lack of funds; poverty due to medical expenses as well as to the need to "spend down" any savings to near zero in order to receive Medicaid; and the inability to obtain insurance to cover medical and funeral expenses.

Physically, AIDS patients face loss of sex drive (usually temporary), extreme weight loss, the pain and disfigurement of sores and blisters, physical weakness, and incapacitation. For many AIDS patients, young men in the prime of life with active social and professional lives, these conditions are extremely disheartening. Along with the loss of physical vitality, AIDS robs these people of their self-esteem, their means of identifying themselves within the society. In addition, AIDS patients lose their identity as financial entities; no loans or home mortgages are possible if their diagnosis is known.

A patient's reaction to an AIDS diagnosis varies, but several common reactions are shock, denial, guilt, fear, anger, sadness, and depression, not necessarily in this order. The individual often feels shunned by society and may feel unclean and unworthy.

The patient's fears are often many: fear of death and dying, fear of lifestyle exposure, fear of loss of physical attractiveness, fear of social isolation, fear of dying alone and unwanted on the street.

The guilt many AIDS patients feel often stems from internal conflicts about lifestyle, conflicts usually reawakened by renewed contact with their biological families. AIDS patients who have infected their lovers feel a burden of guilt for this too. Intentionally and unintentionally, caregivers may reinforce this guilt.

Issues of dependency arise. If the disease progresses, patients lose autonomy and must rely upon strangers—a difficult issue for young, previously active people. Loss of positive body image, loss of social support, and loss of income contribute to the concern.

Finally, there are the major concerns and confusion regarding the course of the disease and the medical options available. Patients are accustomed to receiving accurate information about disease. However, patients with AIDS face an absence of concrete information, and may find that doctors and health care workers are themselves unsure about the course of the disease. Some of these professionals may be experiencing fear and helplessness as they struggle with the current limitations of medicine.

Faced with this uncertainty, many patients try to bargain. Patients wish to be told that if they perform some function—exercise right, eat right, "be good," stop smoking—then the disease will go away. Bargaining may be a way of avoiding the situation and the need to make realistic decisions. Many patients turn away from the hopelessness they see in their caregivers' eyes, and seek out experimental or quack treatments that quickly deplete their financial resources. The uncertainty of the medical staff also fuels the patients' anger, since they may believe, rightly or wrongly, that not everything possible is being done on their behalf. Simmering anger at the person who infected them, or at family members who have reappeared in their lives, is often present. Anger is often directed at the government. Patients who contracted AIDS via blood transfusions are particularly angry.

The depression associated with AIDS is often major. Depression is a natural reaction to discovering that one has a noncurable disease and may soon die. This depression conforms to standard psychological definitions. Depression may also be a physiological part of the syndrome, caused by HIV or an opportunistic infection.

Some patients evolve into a stage of acceptance and are able to function without undue psychological impairment. They may adopt healthier lifestyles, avoid risk, and regain their normal composure. Some patients are able to reconcile their relationships with parents, family, and friends. In some cases, however, the acceptance is not healthy. Patients may give up, saying, "Some of us make it, some of us don't," and may forego helpful treatment.

Some patients feel a certain relief on diagnosis. Typically, these patients have been feeling ill for an extended period of time. Diagnosis may have been a long, painful, frightening experience. The diagnosis simply confirms their worst suspicions.

Intimate relationships tend to polarize after diagnosis. There is a tendency for AIDS patients and their lovers either to bond more closely or to separate entirely.

Psychiatric Symptoms of AIDS

The psychiatric symptoms common to HIV infection stem from two possible sources: emotional reaction to AIDS diagnosis and physical damage of central nervous system tissue by HIV infection or opportunistic infections. Early in the AIDS epidemic, many unfortunate patients experiencing delirium or dementia were chastised by caregivers for being loud, unruly, and uncooperative when, in reality, this inappropriate behavior was the result of organic damage to the brain or central nervous system. When AIDS patients exhibit inappropriate behavior, organic disorders should be suspected although emotional distress may also be the cause.

Depression, fatigue, confusion, apathy, lack of appetite, loss of weight, loss of sex drive, and night sweats may be the initial symptoms of AIDS, or may be purely psychological reactions to stress. In an individual worried about being HIV-infected, emotional distress can trigger somatic symptoms which mimic AIDS, thus fueling additional emotional distress. These patients often experience chronic anxiety, characterized by panic attacks, fast heart beat, agitation, inability to eat, phobias, insomnia, and hypochondrias.

The psychiatric symptoms of AIDS may be classified into two groups: the depression cluster and the psychotic cluster.

The Depression Cluster. The depression cluster is characterized by apathy and loss of interest in typical activities, refusing to eat, extreme passivity, social withdrawal, hypochondria, fatigue, anxiety, subtle personality changes, sleeping too much, forgetfulness, impaired concentration, and perhaps impairment of fine movement psychomotor activities. These symptoms may be quite mild.

The Psychotic Cluster. The onset of the psychotic cluster is usually more abrupt and noticeable. The psychotic cluster may include major depression as well as the psychotic components. A psychosis is an emotional or behavioral problem that interferes with normal social functioning. Psychotic disorders include schizophrenic-like personality changes, acute paranoia, and the excessive excitement of mania. Symptoms of these disorders include confusion, rambling and repetitive speech, psychomotor agitation, hallucinations, and delusional and grandiose thinking.

Many of these symptoms can be loosely categorized under the term *delirium*. Delirium occurs in more than 50 percent of AIDS patients, according to some reports. Delirium generally has an organic basis and can often be alleviated with drug treatments.

The psychotic cluster often occurs during an acute medical crisis. However, these conditions may precede, follow, or coincide with the symptoms of the depression cluster.

The Issue of Denial. In denial, an individual simply pretends that a problem does not exist. Denial is probably the most common psychological defense in our society. Limited experimental evidence suggests that denial may offer some immunological benefit. However, denial may also delay the quest for medical evaluation and treatment. It is suggested that denial be tolerated unless it interferes with medical treatment or places others at risk.

Denial often exists long before an individual seeks medical or psychological help. Denial also hampers educational efforts, and this must be taken into consideration. When people say "I just don't want to deal with this AIDS stuff," or "I've heard enough about this AIDS thing," this may be a sign that counseling is necessary. Fear-inducing anti-AIDS campaigns, the most common format used, probably do not promote long-term healthy behaviors.

Typical Progression. The 2- to 4-month period following the diagnosis of AIDS is one of intense emotional turmoil, often followed by a period of relative quiescence. Individuals may find comfort in the belief that they will be one of the long-term survivors.

The next psychological crisis can be triggered by the appearance of an opportunistic infection or hospitalization. Survival beliefs may be replaced by the belief that they will die. At this point, psychological symptoms may develop rapidly or existing symptoms become worse.

Evaluation. Interviews and standard psychological tests can be used to determine the cognitive and emotional status of the individual. Ongoing evaluations should be done as conditions change.

Treatment. Standard psychotherapeutic drug treatment is successful in treating AIDS patients, although they seem to be unusually sensitive to drugs and require smaller doses than other patients. The emotional components of distress can be handled by sympathetic counselors. (See the section below on counseling.)

Emotions and the Immune System

Emotions affect general health and immune system function. In a small study of breast cancer patients, the patients with "a fighting spirit" survived longer than patients who acted helpless, hopeless, and stoical. The mechanisms of survival are not understood. Perhaps emotions trigger immune response which enhance or weaken resistance to cancer.

An interesting study on homosexual men provides additional evidence that emotions affect the immune system. In a large group of homosexual men who had tested negative for HIV, men who believed that they had lymphadenopathy syndrome (LAS) had lower immune function, measured by T-helpers to T-suppressor ratios, than men who did not believe they had LAS. T-cell ratios correlated with these beliefs and not with the presence of LAS.

Stress-Reduction Techniques. Relaxation techniques may also alter the function of the immune system. In a group of elderly people, relaxation techniques practiced three times weekly raised natural killer cell (NK) activity.

AIDS Phobia

A phobia is an irrational fear of something, where the fear exceeds reasonable concern. Fear is HIV's best weapon. Fear prevents rational behavior and interferes with conscious infection control and the development of a reasonable public health policy. Fear grows in an atmosphere of ignorance, where accurate information is not available. Phobias may grow out of fears, and are usually caused by the transference of anxieties from other concerns to one particular issue.

The public's fear of AIDS is well demonstrated: After years of growth, blood donations to the Red Cross dropped 5 percent in 1983; employees have fled work sites shared with HIV-infected people; and schools have become legal battlegrounds on AIDS-related issues. The school situation perhaps best illustrates the transference of fears. A combination of unreliable information about AIDS, a growing distrust of authorities, and a feeling of loss of control over personal issues are probably fueling the parental overreactions to the presence of HIV-infected children in the schools.

Physical symptoms of AIDS phobia are now being seen by doctors. People break out with herpes blisters and become heavily depressed and suicidal. Unfaithful married men experience depression, anxiety, weight loss, and fatigue, symptoms similar to the initial symptoms of AIDS. In fact some individuals have been diagnosed with "pseudo-AIDS," because their emotional distress has caused symptoms mimicking AIDS.

In people at high risk for HIV infection, and in people who test positive (some of whom are false-positive), AIDS phobia can take a deadly turn. Many of these people experience symptoms which may be pseudo-AIDS or may be the initial symptoms of AIDS itself. In either case, suicide is a real risk.

Testing

Testing Issues. When the AIDS blood test was first developed, there was questionable value in being tested. The psychological impact of testing positive can be devastating, and before AZT no treatment could offer a counterbalance. To know was to lose hope. Considering that denial may offer an immunological benefit, in the past it may have been better for a person at high risk to remain ignorant of his or her true status, assuming that the person took precautions not to transmit HIV.

Now, AZT offers the seropositive person some hope. AZT provides individuals with a reason to learn their HIV status. With HIV infection, as with so many other medical conditions, early detection and early treatment may lead to better clinical outcome or control. One current issue is whether to administer AZT to seropositive individuals who have no symptoms of AIDS.

Individuals who are young, nonwhite, with limited education are less likely to want to know their HIV status. Studies suggest that, for a number of reasons, healthier behaviors (nonsmoking, health maintenance, etc.) are more likely to be practiced by high-income individuals. These behavioral differences must be overcome through education and peer pressure.

Testing and Behavior. Test results can be a strong motivator for behavioral change. Statistically, the knowledge of being seropositive seems to lead to less risky behavior. However, in seronegative individuals, some studies indicate that test results encourage adverse sexual behavior. Other studies suggest that test results do improve the behavior of seronegatives, but to a lesser extent than seropositives.

Pre-Test Counseling. Prior to testing, individuals need to be counseled and given written information explaining the test results and instructions about sexual hygiene, safer sex practices, and infection control. If counseling services are not available at the facility, then the individual should be referred to another resource.

Post-Test Counseling. When people receive their test results, counseling must be available. The psychological impact of a seropositive test is extreme. Immediate counseling must be available before the individual leaves the facility; a follow-up appointment with an appropriate counselor should be made. There is a risk of suicide. If the facility does not have counseling services available, then the facility should not be administering the test. The way in which a seropositive result is presented can be crucial, particularly in the time period between the initial ELISA test and the confirmatory Western blot test.

Seronegative individuals should again receive information on sexual hygiene, safer sex, infection control procedures, and may want to be referred to counseling for compulsive behavioral problems or to relevant support groups. Test results alone are not effective in promoting safer behavior in seronegatives. People should be discouraged from using testing as a measure of their health status. A seronegative result does not mean that high-risk activities are safe.

Changing High-Risk Behavior

The switch from high-risk to low-risk activities is not easy for everyone. A person accustomed to high-risk behaviors has to learn a new set of social and sexual skills, for instance, how to negotiate safe sex agreements. Caution may run counter to deeply ingrained compulsive behaviors.

Studies of selected homosexual male populations report a reduction in high-risk sexual activities such as multiple anonymous sex partners and receptive anal intercourse. Evidence supports these self-reported findings. For example, in some areas where AIDS is common, there have been decreases in the number of cases of anal gonorrhea among homosexual men. This decrease could indicate a decrease in anal intercourse or a decrease in unprotected anal intercourse. These changes vary according to region. Where AIDS is common, many homosexual men report a reduction of high-risk sexual activities. However, in other regions where AIDS is not common, the high-risk practices seem to be continuing.

Even in regions where AIDS is common, the ability of an individual to avoid high-risk behaviors varies. Studies performed at the University of Michigan found that AIDS-related knowledge, self-perceived risk, actual degree of risk, and social network were factors affecting the avoidance of high-risk behavior. These researchers found that increased knowledge led to healthier behavior. The number of anonymous sexual contacts was reduced, anal intercourse was avoided, and condoms were used during sexual intercourse. Consequently, these researchers suggest that education alone gives the greatest return on behavior improvement. This suggestion is supported by the reported effectiveness of education among homosexuals in high-risk cities. Peer groups serve an important educational function. The researchers emphasize the role of gay organizations and social networks in promoting risk reduction.

Unfortunately, these researchers found that some of the individuals at highest risk were least able to alter their behavior. Some of the factors involved were denial and control. Denial can cause people to misinterpret information. High-risk individuals who continue high-risk activities tend to distort epidemiological evidence and exclude themselves from statistical risk. They are not realistic in the matter of self-perceived risk. People's perceptions of the personal control they have over the events in their lives are thought to be related to compulsive behavior. Many aspects of AIDS make it seem to be beyond personal control, for example, the long incubation period, the uncertainty of prognosis, and the uncertainty of medical professionals. Researchers found that a high degree of personal helplessness and a high self-perceived personal health risk, combined, were statistically linked to adverse sexual behaviors. For compulsive individuals focused on "quick-fix" rewards, avoidance of high-risk behavior seems beyond their personal abilities. These individuals find implausible excuses such as "If I haven't got it already, I won't," and "I take plenty of vitamins and exercise regularly," or rely on faith and mysticism instead of changing their behavior.

Figure 18: Important Information for Seropositive People.

- The HIV antibody does not grant immunity.
- The long-term prognosis of having the HIV antibody is unknown.
- Asymptomatic individuals probably are able to transmit HIV.
- Not donate blood, plasma, body organs, tissue or sperm for use in humans.
- Not share toothbrushes, razors, and other possibly blood-contaminated instruments with other people.
- Inform their sex partner(s) of their seropositive status.
- Inform medical and dental caregivers of their seropositivity.
- How to prevent sexual transmission.
- How to handle blood accidents.
- The current information on disease progression.
- Where to receive additional counseling.

Counseling

Ideally, counseling should reduce anxiety, alleviate depression, lessen self-destructive impulses, help the patient cope with physical stresses and limitations, and perhaps provide a pathway for reconciliation with friends and family, if necessary. Counseling should be provided in terms and language that the client understands and should progress at a speed that is comfortable for the client. The counselor should aid the patient by reinforcing the patient's own positive coping methods and by encouraging the patient to recall successful responses to previous stressful events. These responses can be used as guidelines for coping with the current situation.

Counselors must be well informed about AIDS, including the physical, neurological, and psychiatric symptoms. Mental health professionals should be able to recognize the common psychological complications of AIDS, such as anxiety, depression, obsessive and compulsive behaviors, neurological disorders, and suicide risk. In addition to maintaining close contact with medical staff, counselors should be aware of local services and resources available for their clients. These include AIDS service organizations; local support groups; city, state, county, and federal agencies; visiting nurses associations; local hospices; and volunteer and religious organizations.

Counselors must watch their own emotional responses. According to some reports, therapists are prone to develop fears of personal invasion, particularly as the client-patient relationship develops. Many therapists feel an excessive need to become experts on AIDS in an effort to counter their own feelings of helplessness. Some overwhelmed therapists may prematurely refer the patient to self-help groups, triggering feelings of rejection and abandonment in the patient.

High-Risk Individuals. Many of the individuals at high risk for HIV infection may have prejudices against mental health professionals. Some homosexuals and drug addicts may feel that the counselor has prejudged them, and sees only a "bad" stereotype. This fear is not without foundation. Counselors must assess their own fears and attitudes related to AIDS, such as fear of contagion and of people who practice high-risk activities, such as homosexuals and IV drug users.

Gay-affirmative therapists attempt to alter the internalized negative feelings felt by some homosexuals, and encourage the expression of homosexual feelings and safe forms of sexual expression.

A common belief of counselors is that traditional practices will not work with AIDS patients, because of the extremity of their distress. In actuality, counselors experienced with AIDS patients report that traditional practices, with some modifications and allowances for value differences, do help. A poll of AIDS patients revealed that, although they may have received an abundance of medical attention and information, they may not have anybody with whom to share their intimate concerns. Common issues are psychotherapy itself, life and death, personal limits, finding meaning in life, loneliness, helplessness, the illness and death of friends, and conflicts regarding a chosen lifestyle.

Seropositive Individuals. Seropositive people need immediate social and psychological counseling. Suicide risk is high following a seropositive test result. People need to be immediately linked to a lifeline, given the name and number of an appropriate counselor who can help them through the emotional crisis. They must be encouraged to inform their sexual partners of their seropositive status and to practice infection control in their sexual, domestic, occupational, social, and recreational settings.

Seropositive individuals need to come to terms both with their high-risk behaviors and the alterations necessary for infection control. Seropositive individuals need education on all aspects of AIDS, and need to be encouraged to make overall lifestyle improvements to boost their health status, such as improving diet, sleep and exercise regimens, eliminating drugs and alcohol, avoiding STDs and other infectious diseases, avoiding undue stress, and learning alternative stress-reduction techniques.

For obvious reasons, these individuals may have obsessional thoughts about death and dying. Concentration on the job or at home may be poor; relationships with other people may become strained.

Many asymptomatic individuals develop acute psychological symptoms, such as panic attacks, generalized anxiety, and physical reactions which mimic AIDS. Characteristic episodes center on unfounded beliefs that the person has developed AIDS and is dying, accompanied by repeated visits to emergency rooms, AIDS screening clinics, and the offices of mental health professionals. Counselors must watch for distortion of information and misinterpretation of facts on the part of the client.

The neurological symptoms of AIDS can precede the physical symptoms and may not be apparent without neuropsychiatric testing. Monitoring should be ongoing.

It is suggested that seropositive individuals can benefit from stress inoculation (administering manageable doses of stress) and problem-solving techniques. Experienced counselors suggest that clarification, verbalizing and acting out, palliative relaxation techniques, cognitive appraisal, cognitive reframing, and support are effective if the therapist allows the patient the regression naturally associated with the sick role. A temporary regression to a more dependent state might be expected and need not necessarily be viewed as an individual characteristic.

To help overcome negative-self attitudes, the therapist can ally with the patient and help reduce inappropriate sexual and other behavior. By stating at the outset that a goal of therapy is to help the client be responsible, the therapist addresses the individual's healthier ego functions. The patient's guilt of being infected can be offset by a pride in not infecting others. A sense of mastery over present behavior can be important when faced with the uncertainty of HIV infection.

Seropositive Individuals with Symptoms. The development of clinical symptoms and opportunistic infections in a seropositive person greatly increases the stress on individuals. The psychological duress increases with the added burdens of disfigurement, the inability to work or socialize, and perhaps hospitalization. Extreme withdrawal, depression, and chronic anxiety may result. All these emotional states may be immunosuppressive. Suicide risk is at its peak.

More than ever, the individual needs to be encouraged to attend support groups. Many refuse to attend before symptoms develop because they prefer to deny their illness and do not wish to reveal their HIV status or problematic behaviors. Polls reveal that very few seropositive and ill people currently use community and psychiatric services.

When and if the client is ready, this may be the time to begin discussion of the possible course of the disease and the medical options available. One topic might be the use of life-sustaining treatment, although this might also be left to the attending physician. Many patients have considered this issue.

If therapy is just beginning at this point, experienced counselors suggest focusing on the physical symptoms, working on the acceptance of physical disorders, and recognizing and establishing physical limits. The counselor can then ascertain what the client thinks is important. The client may benefit from the release of stress by verbalizing or acting out from therapeutic suggestion.

AIDS. When the client develops AIDS, he or she may be physically and emotionally overwhelmed by the disease and the need to make decisions. If the individual's health continues to decline, terminal psychological techniques can aid in preparing for death. Reportedly, people who are dying desire and benefit from psychotherapy. The therapist can aid with frequent visits and nonverbal communications of support and care. Therapy allows the patient to express deep-seated, often conflicting emotions and fears.

Sexual Partners. The sexual partners of seropositive people need education and support. These individuals must come to terms with their fear of infection and the changes that infection control introduces into their lives. Also, these individuals must contend with their own HIV status, and must make de-

Figure 19: Suggested Support Groups

- For homosexual men concerned about AIDS.
- For seropositive people.
- For seropositive people with symptoms.
- For AIDS patients in the hospital.
- For sexually compulsive homosexual and/or bisexual men.
- For sexually compulsive heterosexuals.
- For married, bisexual men.
- For IV drug users.
- For male, female, and teenage prostitutes.
- For bereaved family and friends.

cisions concerning testing. The AIDS patient may blame the partner, or vice versa, for the presence of the disease. Partners may be dealing with the care of the AIDS patient and with the eventual death of that person.

Family and Friends. If the AIDS patient is a member of a socially stigmatized group, he or she may be estranged from biological family. The reintroduction of this family into the life of the patient may reawaken many of the patient's internal and external conflicts. In the case of homosexual patients, the biological family often blames the patient's sexual partner for the disease. Sometimes mothers of patients have a tendency to assume responsibility for the patient's situation.

When assessing the patient's needs, an accompanying assessment of the needs of the patient's friends and family is desirable, since the psychological impact of family issues can adversely affect the patient.

Homosexual relationships are not legally sanctioned, though homosexual "common law" marriages may be emotionally and financially binding. In some instances, the partners of AIDS patients have lost financial support and been barred from the hospital by the patient's biological families. Biological families are often legally permitted to make medical decisions should the patient become mentally incompetent and to carry out funeral arrangements, perhaps barring the partner from that as well.

If the patient's biological family is inadequate or hostile, a patient advocate can be legally assigned to carry out the patient's wishes, should the patient become incompetent.

Support Groups. Figure 19 lists the suggested populations that might benefit from peer support groups. Support groups are particularly necessary for seropositive and symptomatic people. Otherwise isolation and subsequent withdrawal and depression result. Sometimes these groups are totally casual; sometimes they benefit from professional guidance. Many AIDS service organizations sponsor these types of support groups, open to all types of individuals. Additional volunteer support groups are being formed by a number of concerned religious and social organizations.

9. Death with Dignity

Death may not be the inevitable result of HIV infection, particularly as more suitable anti-HIV drugs become available, and as medical professionals learn better how to fine-tune therapy in order to control opportunistic infections and keep secondary effects within limits.

However, at some point in the syndrome, death and preparation for death are topics of concern that should be discussed. Discussions should take place between the patient and the appropriate caregivers. Such discussion might also benefit family members. Quite often, the patient knows when death is near, as does the family. However, seeking to protect each other, both often prefer to pretend that everything is all right.

Life-Sustaining Procedures

Life-sustaining procedures use mechanical devices to keep the patient alive who would otherwise die. By the time life-sustaining equipment is used, the patient has usually lost consciousness and has virtually no hope of returning to consciousness or to a normal, wakeful, healthy state.

It is best for individual patients to decide whether they desire life-sustaining treatment or whether resuscitation should be attempted if their hearts stop beating.

AIDS patients rarely broach the subject with their attending physicians. Physicians are also reluctant to discuss life-sustaining treatment with patients. Physicians fear that patients may interpret such discussions as surrender on the part of the physicians. Rather than discuss the options, some physicians simply default to common practice.

A tendency exists for patients to overestimate the effects of life-sustaining treatment. Caregivers must watch for this distortion.

For physicians, experience may be the best guide as to when life-sustaining treatment needs to be discussed and the options described. Hospital policy may also dictate protocol. When explaining life-sustaining options, the physician must stress that care and the fight for life will continue. In some hospitals, physicians discuss "Do-Not-Resuscitate" orders within 72 hours of hospitalization, to avoid rushed and haphazard discussions later.

Patient Advocate

A patient advocate is an individual chosen to speak in the patient's stead should the patient become mentally incompetent or physically unable to communicate. The patient advocate can become legally entitled to make financial and medical decisions on the patient's behalf. Unless other arrangements are made, these legal powers revert to the patient's biological family. The term *patient advocate* has no legal definition, but its use has been adopted by a number of AIDS service organizations.

Several methods allow patients to pass on legal rights, depending on the state. First, patients can nominate another individual to be their guardian or conservator. A court appearance is necessary for this procedure.

Some states allow patients to grant power of attorney to a chosen individual, allowing this individual to make financial or medical decisions for the patient. Special conditions or limitations may be written into the power of attorney.

In some states a "living will" can instruct physicians to remove artificial life-sustaining systems. Living wills can be problematic since they are inflexible, sometimes ambiguous, and not necessarily legally binding.

An "inter vivos trust" enables patients to pass financial decisions to other individuals.

All of these documents can be revoked at any time should patients choose to make their own decisions.

As much as possible, the patient advocate should be present at all major medical discussions between patient and caregivers; this builds the advocate's knowledge of the patient's medical picture and of the patient's desires. The patient advocate may be called upon to use this knowledge to interpret the patient's wishes and make final medical decisions regarding resuscitation and other life-sustaining medical options.

Hospices

Hospices are care centers specifically designed for dying patients, emphasizing practical pain-lessening care and emotional support for patients and the patient's loved ones. Generally, hospices have interdisciplinary nursing teams and may utilize community volunteers. Historically, hospices have provided care for terminal cancer patients.

Hospices differ in approaches and in the types of patients they accept; for example, some hospices only accept cancer patients. As a requirement for some hospices, the patient must acknowledge that he or she is going to die. Some hospices are affiliated with only one hospital, thus limiting the patient's choice of physicians. Some continue to offer care even after insurance coverage is exhausted; those receiving Medicare funds are, reportedly, not allowed to terminate care. Some administer emotional care and bereavement counseling for survivors on a continuing basis. When considering a hospice, patients should be sure to clarify the options.

Information on hospices may be obtained from the National Cancer Institute (1-800-4-CANCER), AIDS service organizations, local hospitals, visiting nurses associations, and, perhaps, from local religious organizations.

Dying at Home

Some patients may wish to die at home, attended by visiting nurses and loved ones. This option is not advised for everyone, as it places an exceptional demand on the emotional resources of the patient's family and friends. Caring for AIDS patients in the home provides an alternative to hospitalization, a more comforting environment for some patients, and potentially reduces the cost of care. The reduction in cost usually stems from use of volunteer labor.

All caregivers in the home should be trained in the basic patient care procedures, in HIV transmission precautions, such as hand-washing, glove procedures, etc. Caregivers, particularly volunteers, should receive some counseling on the emotional aspects of caring for AIDS patients, and, ideally, should have a support group available.

Euthanasia

Euthanasia means "painless death." In a sense, physicians provide dying patients with "passive" euthanasia by not hooking them up to life-sustaining equipment. "Active" euthanasia is practiced in the Netherlands, where physicians are allowed to inject lethal drugs into terminally ill patients. A strict protocol exists. In the past cancer patients have usually been involved; apparently, Dutch AIDS patients will also have this option available to them.

The Hemlock Society. The Hemlock Society is an educational organization which promotes the option of rational, voluntary euthanasia. Euthanasia is defined by the Hemlock Society as the willful act of dying on the part of individuals with incurable diseases. The founders of the Hemlock Society were men and women whose spouses died of cancer. However, AIDS may no longer be incurable, depending on the long-term effects of AZT and other drugs as they become available.

Generally, suicide is not a crime; however, it is a crime to help another person to commit suicide.

Rational euthanasia is voluntary and performed by the patient who is incurable and mentally competent, who probably has suffered irreversible major bodily damage, and who looks forward to assured death after much additional suffering.

During HIV infection, the patient may not be rational, due to organic brain damage, even when no other clinical symptoms are evident; suicide attempts are likely to be irrational. Individuals tend to attempt suicide soon after being notified of seropositivity, after the first bout of opportunistic infections or during or after their first round of hospitalization.

The Hemlock Society publishes a book entitled *Let Me Die Before I Wake*. A guide to "self-deliverance," this book tells the stories of terminally ill patients who have sought to end their lives, illustrates the kinds of decisions someone considering this option must make, and gives the details of "successful" methods, typically using drugs.

For more information, call the Hemlock Society at (213) 391-1871, or write to P.O. Box 66218, Los Angeles, CA 90066.

10. Preventing AIDS

Ending or controlling the AIDS epidemic requires action on both individual and societal levels. Each individual must, wherever possible, take precautions to avoid HIV infection. As a society we must ensure that every individual receives adequate education about AIDS and the physical, social, and emotional aspects of sexual activity. In addition, society must make allowances for individuals not capable of taking care of themselves and provide the necessary social support structures.

All members of society must participate in this education—not just people in the high-risk groups. Disease seeks any opportunity to advance and disregards any human definitions of social organization. Until more information is available about the extent of AIDS in the general population, we should pretend that we are all infected and take the appropriate precautions.

Sexual Hygiene

Sex does not cause AIDS. Sex does not cause disease, unless one practices it beyond the body's limits of endurance. Through certain sexual acts, the Human Immunodeficiency Virus (HIV) may be passed from one person to another. In most instances, the *exchange or transference of bodily fluids* between sexual partners is responsible for the transmission of HIV. Most likely, HIV-infected cells transmit infection from one person to another, not cell-free viruses. Semen and blood are probably the major culprits; feces, urine, mother's milk, and vaginal and cervical secretions are probably secondary culprits. Saliva and tears transmit HIV rarely, if ever.

Hygiene is the practice of following certain health rules. In the age of AIDS, *sexual hygiene* means avoiding the exchange of bodily fluids and secretions during sexual activity. Strictly speaking, semen, vaginal and cervical secretions, blood, urine, feces, saliva, tears, and mother's milk from one person should not be placed into the mouth, nose, eyes, ears, vagina, anus, or open wounds (even microscopic) of another person. Hopefully, sexual hygiene will prevent HIV transmission and the transmission of other STDs, by using both physical and behavioral barriers.

Physical and behavioral barriers are used to reduce the transmission of HIV and other STDs. Some degree of risk is always present. Combined use of proper barrier techniques can reduce the risk of catching AIDS or other STDs very close to zero.

Condoms

Condom use may reduce the risk of contracting AIDS or an HIV infection, as indicated by both laboratory and clinical studies. Condoms should be used to prevent the exchange of bodily fluids during vaginal or anal intercourse or fellatio (mouth-penis contact). Condoms are also used to prevent environmental contamination by contaminated sperm. People should be prepared in advance because sexual passion often interferes with clear thinking.

Condoms are a physical barrier, preventing contact between the tissues and fluids of one sexual partner and the tissues and fluids of the other. Condoms are not perfect barriers; they can have invisible pinholes or cracks, and, under the stress of use, can break open or slip off. Spermicide or contraceptive jelly should accompany condom use. See below.

Reportedly, condom failure is usually due to human factors, rather than to the mechanical failure of the condom's material. Generally, human failure means: (1) failure to use a condom; (2) failure to use condoms *all the time*; (3) failure to use a condom at the right time; (4) failure to lubricate the condom properly; or (5) spillage of semen from the condom into a partner's body cavity because of improper condom handling. (See Figure 20 on condom use.)

Most condoms are made of *latex*, basically a form of rubber. Approximately 1 percent of condoms sold are *natural*, made of the "skin" which lines sheep's intestines. Some people choose natural condoms, believing them to be more "sensitive" than latex or because they are allergic to latex, condom dyes, or other additives. Latex condoms are more resistant to leakage than natural condoms, as evidenced by laboratory experiments.

Condoms vary in size and width, and generally these factors vary slightly from nation to nation. When going on vacation, it is best to bring your own along with you.

Condom Efficiency. Most information on condom efficiency comes from pregnancy prevention studies. Based on one fairly large study, the statistical risk of pregnancy due to condom failure is 1 pregnancy in 10,000 uses. Since the chance of pregnancy is 2 to 4 percent following injection of semen, a pregnancy rate of 1 in 10,000 means that there were 50 to 100 condom failures resulting in semen injection. A human female can only be impregnated during approximately 48 hours each menstrual cycle. A viral agent is, presumably, always present and always able to infect upon exposure, although exposure does not always result in infection.

In this condom study, the failure rate of the condoms was between 0.25 and 0.5 percent. However, other studies estimate failure rates to be between 4 and 36 percent (between 4 and 36 failures per 100 uses). A significant difference in failure rate exists among brands.

Brands. Different brands of condoms have differing failure rates or rates of leakage. All commercially manufactured condoms must pass the approval of the Food and Drug Administration (FDA), but there is a wide range of quality. Researchers suggest avoiding "boutique" brands because the manufacturing and quality control techniques may not be on a par with those of the major condom manufacturers.

With the advent of AIDS, many new types of condoms supposedly designed for anal intercourse have been marketed. Most claims have not been substantiated by experimental studies.

In one mechanical (nonhuman) experiment, the following brands were tested and found to retain the HIV virus: Trojan ENZ, Trojan ENZ Lubricated, Fourex

Figure 20: Condom Use

When:	Use condom for oral, anal, and vaginal sex. Use every single time. Put on condom as soon as erection occurs or before pre-ejaculatory fluid appears on tip of penis. Be prepared in advance; sexual passion often interferes with clear thinking. Practice condom use beforehand. Practice makes perfect.
Removing Condom From Package:	Carefully inspect package for holes, cracks, and damage. Discard condom if package is open. Carefully open the package to avoid damaging the condom. Inspect condom for holes, cracks, and signs of aging, dryness, or brittleness. Discard if necessary.
Putting on the Condom:	Leave condom rolled up. Note that condom unrolls only one way. If the wrong side of condom becomes contaminated with moisture from penis, discard condom. With the thumb and finger of one hand, gently squeeze and hold the condom tip. Then, place condom over tip of penis, and unroll condom over full length of penis with the other hand. Squeezing the condom tip ensures that no air remains in tip, leaving room for semen. When unrolling condom down shaft of penis, take care to expell all air. Air bubbles can cause the condom to break. As condom nears base of penis, brush pubic hair towards base of penis. This prevents the pubic hair from becoming painfully entangled in the condom. Unroll condom to base of penis.
Lubrication:	It is best to lubricate the condom. Inadequate lubrication is suspected to be a major cause of condom breakage. Water-based lubricants, non-allergenic surgical lubricants (such as K-Y Jelly), and contraceptive jellies and foams are OK to use and are available in pharmacies and sex specialty shops. Read the label. DO NOT use petroleum-based lubricants, such as Petroleum Jelly. DO NOT use saliva, cooking oil, or cold cream. Saliva may contain germs. Petroleum-based substances dissolve latex. Avoid over-long exposure of condom to spermicides and contraceptive creams. No problem should develop during the timespan of normal use.

Figure 20: Condom Use (Continued)

Ejaculation:	After male ejaculation, body movement should stop or be reduced to the absolute minimum. Once the inside of the condom becomes wet, the condom can easily slip off and spill its contents inside the receptive partner. At this point, check with the hand to make sure that the condom is securely in place.
Penis Withdrawal From Partner:	Hold onto base of condom when withdrawing penis, otherwise it is likely to slip off and spill its contents into receptive partner. Before removing condom, brush pubic hair out of the vicinity. Roll condom up shaft of penis, then slide condom off without spilling contents.
Disposal:	High risk individuals should take care in disposing of condoms. Semen is a potentially contaminated substance. Condoms might be disposed of in a bedside container of 1 part bleach and 10 parts water. Most toilet systems can handle condoms.
Storage:	Condoms should not be exposed to extremes of hot or cold. Condoms should be stored somewhere near room temperature. DO NOT store condoms in sunlight. DO NOT expose condoms with windows in the package to flourescent light. DO NOT store condoms in the glove boxes of cars. The coolest place in a car is under the front seats. Wallets are not a good place for condoms: replace them regularly if carried there.
Emergency:	Keep a can of contraceptive foam handy. Should a condom fail or semen spillage occur, fill the vagina with contraceptive or spermicidal foam. Spermicides having nonoxynol-9 or benzalkonium chloride have anti-HIV action. Spermicides and contraceptive foams are not FDA approved for use in the anus. Douching has a statistical risk of increasing HIV infection, according to studies of anal intercourse among homosexual males.
Reuse:	Never reuse a condom.

lubricated (natural), Ramses Extra, and Skinless Skin (synthetic skin). These products may or may not retain HIV or fluids during actual use, and a number of other condom products may or may not be more efficient.

Manufacturer Testing. Most manufacturers claim to check each condom individually. Generally this is done by placing the condom over a metal penisform and passing an electrical charge through it. If any hole is present in the condom, then the electricity will burn a wider hole through it. Additionally, condoms are selected randomly and filled with water.

Reportedly, the FDA also checks batches of condoms from manufacturers. Allegedly, current condom quality is partially due to FDA monitoring of condom manufacturing in the 1930s and 1940s.

Viral Challenges. In a number of small studies, condoms have been challenged by viruses to see whether transmission could occur through tiny holes or perforations of the latex—holes perhaps too small to be found by regular testing techniques. In theory, a condom passing the manufacturing tests mentioned above should not allow the passage of HIV or any virus of comparable size. Both electrons and water molecules are smaller than viruses.

In these viral challenges, condoms are placed on a culturing medium (in which a virus will rapidly reproduce), and virus-contaminated fluids are mechanically injected into the condom. In some experiments the condoms were mechanically agitated to simulate the stress of sexual intercourse.

In these tests no escape of HIV out of the condom and onto the medium was found. In addition to HIV, a small mouse virus was tested. No leakage of either virus was found. However, there are other reports that natural condoms leaked herpes viruses where latex condoms did not.

Distribution of Condoms. In the United States, condoms were illegal in many states until the mid-1970s. Associated with condoms were images of premarital sex, prostitution, promiscuity, and disease. In actuality, married couples are primary users of condoms. The image of condoms improved during World War II. The military called them prophylactics, focusing on disease prevention, not birth control, and distributed condoms to all soldiers in the European theater.

In general, access to condoms must be broadened. Any person should be able to obtain a condom at any time. Some homosexual bars distribute free condoms upon request. This practice might be adopted by all establishments promoting social activity, particularly social activities accompanied by drug use. Condoms should be made available through vending machines and retail outlets, particularly around college campuses and, in some settings, junior and senior high schools. Ideally, in addition to condom distribution, targeted individuals should receive appropriate education on condom use and sexual hygiene, and have access to the necessary professional, medical, and psychological services.

Other Physical Barriers

Diaphragms. Diaphragms may reduce the risk of transmitting or catching HIV, particularly if menstrual bleeding is taking place. Diaphragms are thought to reduce the risk of STD transmission, but few facts are known.

Diaphragms reduce the risk of pregnancy by physically covering the cervix, the doorway to the uterus, so that sperm is not able to enter. Menstrual bleeding originates in the uterus when the internal surface of the uterus is shed each month. Blood is known to contain HIV; menstrual blood may also contain HIV. A female's ability to transmit HIV may or may not depend on menstrual bleeding.

Whereas condoms prevent any physical contact between sexual partners, diaphragms do not cover all the tissues inside a woman's vagina. Diaphragms should be cleaned according to the manufacturer's instructions.

Dams. Dams are sheets of latex intended for use in dental surgery; they prevent contamination by covering selected areas. Dams can be used to cover a person's vagina or anus so that oral stimulation can take place with less risk of HIV transmittal between mouth and anus or vagina. Care must be taken not to cross-contaminate the two sides of the dam, or to transport a dam contaminated with vaginal fluids to the anus or vice versa.

Before use, dams must be rinsed to remove a coating of talcum powder. Talcum powder is for external use *only*.

Currently, dams can be bought at dental and medical supply stores. No doubt in a short time they will be available at sex specialty shops and, like condoms, through mail order.

Be sure to dispose of dams safely. Dams should not be flushed down the toilet. After use, dams should be dropped into a container of bleach and water (1 part bleach, 9 parts water) for at least 10 minutes before disposal.

Contraceptive Jellies and Spermicides. Contraceptive jellies or spermicides (sperm-killing chemicals) should always be used in conjunction with condoms. By using both condoms and contraceptive chemicals, pregnancy risk approaches zero. Proper use of both should also greatly reduce the risk of HIV transmission.

Some chemicals are now known to inactivate HIV. One chemical available in the United States is *nonoxynol-9,* which is available in spermicidal jellies and foams, some condom lubricants, the tips of some condoms, and perhaps will soon be available as a liquid. Nonoxynol-9 has been tested only for vaginal use and not for its effect on exposed anal tissues.

In a laboratory experiment, nonoxynol-9 was placed in the tips of condoms which were subsequently ruptured. The chemical succeeded in killing two-thirds of the HIV present. Clearly, while offering some protection nonoxynol-9 is not fail-safe.

Another spermicide reportedly effective in killing HIV is *benzalkonium chloride,* a chemical used in contraceptive jellies, creams, and condoms manufactured in France. While it is exported to Canada, Spain, Switzerland, and Africa, benzalkonium chloride has not yet gained FDA approval.

Brands of spermicides and contraceptive jellies differ. If itching or irritation results from use, users should try another brand.

Postcoital Disinfection. *Postcoital* means "after sexual intercourse." Users should always check condoms or diaphragms after sexual intercourse to make sure they were not damaged or displaced. If the integrity of either barrier is in question, then emergency measures may be necessary. One such measure is to fill the vagina with contraceptive foam; a container of foam should be kept on hand for such emergencies. This, however, does not guarantee that neither pregnancy nor infection will result.

Postcoital vaginal douching is commonly believed to reduce the risk of pregnancy and infection. However, in homosexual men, douching was found to increase statistical risk of HIV infection.

Postcoital douching, washing, and irrigation with chemicals have long been practiced as methods of reducing STD transmission. Irrigation of the penis with chemicals after sexual intercourse was common during both world wars. No scientifically controlled studies have been performed on these practices, and so their validity in STD risk reduction is unknown.

Behavioral Barriers

Overcoming Reluctance to Use Physical Barriers. Many people state a number of reasons for not wanting to use physical barriers. Both men and women say barriers interfere with sexual pleasure by interrupting the sex act to put the condom on or the diaphragm in, by reducing the pleasurable sensations of skin-to-skin contact, or by the fact that the presence of the barriers is always noticeable. Opinions vary; some people enjoy condoms, saying the reduced sensation enables them to enjoy the sexual act longer.

Embarrassment is also a key issue in barrier use, beginning with the purchase of condoms and other barriers, and ending with a reluctance to insist on their use. Psychological research indicates that reluctance to raise the issue of condoms often centers around issues of trust. In any case, minor embarrassment must be the cost of low-risk sexual activity in the absence of a long-term monogamous relationship.

The responsibility of purchasing and using barriers should be shared by sexual partners. Each partner should be instructed in how to place the barrier on the other partner, and should exercise this knowledge. Eroticism may be enhanced by making condom or diaphragm placement part of lovemaking.

Selection of Sex Partner. One form of protection against HIV transmission and other STD transmission is careful selection of sexual partners. It may be best to assume that everyone is HIV-infected. In a study of hepatitis B among college students, it was found that people who had more than ten sexual partners were much more likely to have been infected with hepatitis B than people who had had fewer than ten sexual partners. The conclusion of the researchers was that people who are promiscuous are at a higher risk of contracting an STD. *Promiscuous* generally means "having sex with many people"; a more exact definition is "indiscriminate or lacking standards of selection."

It is important to remember that many men and women are bisexual. Not everyone tells the truth all the time. In many college fraternities, a trip to a local area of prostitution has been a traditional initiation rite.

Number of Lifetime Sex Partners. For safety's sake, the number of sex partners should be limited. A high number of sexual partners is the most consistent risk factor associated with catching an HIV infection or other STD, according to statistical research done on homosexual males engaging in unprotected sexual activity. The greater the number of sexual encounters, the greater the chances of encountering HIV. However, one exposure may be sufficient for infection to occur.

If cofactors other than HIV cause AIDS, they too seem to be transmitted sexually.

Drug Use. Some evidence exists that alcohol and other drugs lessen a person's ability to adhere to the rules of sexual hygiene. All drugs affect judgment, especially alcohol, which lowers inhibitions and is known to increase the expression of high-risk behavior. Drugs lower one's mental and emotional barriers.

Experimentation with drugs and sex should not occur at the same time. If sexual activity is expected, people should not consume alcohol or other drugs.

Negotiating Limits. Sexual partners should agree on the limits of sexual activity before such activity begins. Negotiation is a skill which many people need to develop; negotiation of sexual activity is a new, necessary skill.

Unfortunately, people do not necessarily recognize that there are many stages of sexual activity short of intercourse. Intercourse (oral, vaginal, anal) is a high-risk activity which generally should be avoided except between committed sexual partners. Learning satisfying sexual activities other than intercourse may be part of sex education.

Sex Education. Many people do not receive an adequate education regarding sex and reproduction. Almost everyone could learn more. Many books and resources are available to the individual and for use in groups and schools.

Keep in Touch. Since the incubation period of HIV is so long, it is best to keep in touch with all previous sexual partners, perhaps for as long as 15 years. People should keep an up-to-date file of the names and addresses of sexual partners. They should be notified of HIV infection or other STD. As drug treatments become available, HIV infection may fall into the category of most diseases, wherein early detection and early treatment generally lead to an eventual cure.

Household Safety Tips. Razors, toothbrushes, needles, syringes, or any instruments potentially contaminated with blood should not be shared. For instructions in handling blood spills and spills of bodily fluids, see Chapter 19.

When to Stop Using Barriers

If a person is infected with an STD, the risk of transmission to an uninfected partner increases with the number of times they have unprotected sex.

If sexual partners begin a sexual relationship using barriers, then when can they stop using barriers? There is no set rule. Ideally, no sexual partner should have unprotected sex until all partners have been tested for HIV. Such HIV testing should come at least 3 months after the most recent unprotected sexual (or other) exposure, so that antibodies have time to develop. If both partners test negative, then it should be safe to have unprotected sex. Tests are not perfect, however; chances of false-negative or false-positive results do exist.

The sexual and drug use history of one's sexual partners is of great importance when gauging the safety of unprotected sex. It can be difficult to determine what this history is; many people are not completely truthful in regard to sex and drugs.

Currently, HIV is concentrated among certain populations in the United States. The spread of HIV from high-risk groups to the population at large has occurred to an unknown extent. Thus, engaging in unprotected sex with any person increases the risk of contracting HIV.

General Health Issues

Drug Use. If one is HIV-infected, it is a good idea to avoid drugs. As previously mentioned, "poppers" (amyl and butyl nitrites) are statistically associated with the appearance of Kaposi's sarcoma; poppers might even promote Kaposi's sarcoma. Both marijuana and cocaine reportedly impair the immune system. Excessive alcohol consumption is generally unhealthy and promotes malnutrition, which adversely affects the immune system.

Vitamins. People should not take an excessive amount of vitamins unless so directed by a health specialist. Vitamin supplements taken to meet daily requirements are fine. However, excessive iron intake, reportedly practiced by some members of high-risk groups, may promote the growth of bacteria in the intestines and of tumors elsewhere in the body.

Staying Healthy and Improving Hygiene. Each person should try to decrease the size of his or her personal germ pool. The germ pool is the collection of germs a person shares with intimate companions and family members. Personal habits greatly affect the size of the germ pool. Sharing drinking glasses, toothbrushes, bottles, cigarettes, or sex partners with other people increases both the number of germs in the body and obviously the number of people the germs are shared with. Since the development of AIDS may have other cofactors and the replication of HIV may not begin until T-cells are activated by some other germ, avoiding unnecessary germs is a wise idea.

Guidelines: Everyone should drink their own drinks, eat from their own plates, smoke their own cigarettes, etc. People should wash their hands before eating or touching the mouth or eyes. In general, it is best to avoid habits which constantly cause hand-to-face contact, such as smoking or fingernail-biting.

Good health practices apply not only to STD prevention, but also to life in general: Eat right, sleep right, and get enough exercise. Normal exercise helps the lymphatic system function, since the flow of lymph is accomplished by surrounding muscle movement.

It is best to avoid excessive stress whenever possible. Stress-reduction techniques might serve as an alternative to smoking and drinking.

Surgery. In an HIV-infected person, unnecessary surgery should be avoided. Reactions such as anergy (See Figure 11) indicate that the skin's immediate immune defenses are not working well. Thus the individual is more susceptible to infection by the standard, troublesome bacteria present in the operating room environment. (Despite strict precautions, not all microorganisms can be removed from an environment; however, in operating rooms and other sterile environments, the number of bacteria, etc., is so low that body defenses normally have no trouble controlling them.)

Sunlight. The skin is laced with immune cells called Langerhans cells. Langerhans cells capture microbes and present them to T-cells. It seems that Langerhans cells can be damaged by excessive sunlight; therefore, infected individuals may wish to avoid excessive exposure to sunlight.

IV Drug Use Prevention

The use of nonsterile intravenous (IV) drug needles and syringes exposes the user to a number of dangers. Besides HIV, IV drug users often have a history of (1) bacterial infections (Staphylococcus; Streptococcus), both localized at the site of infection and spread throughout the bloodstream; (2) *endocarditis,* the inflammation of membrane lining the heart, usually due to infection by microorganisms; (3) *tetanus,* poisoning by bacterial toxins; and (4) embolisms, wherein particles of air become lodged in blood vessels, blocking blood flow and perhaps resulting in the death of tissues or the death of the person.

The following information should help reduce the risk of problems stemming from HIV and other microorganisms.

Clean Works. Ideally, a hypodermic needle should be used once and discarded. Alternatively, a hypodermic needle, the syringe, and the "cooker" (a container used to heat the drug/water mixture—often a spoon or bottle cap) should be cleaned immediately after every use. All these components, collectively called "the works," can become contaminated with blood. Three cleaning agents are generally available: bleach, ethanol, and isopropyl alcohol.

Bleach is inexpensive and very effective but it slowly corrodes plastic and metal. Bleach must be handled carefully because it is very poisonous to living tissue: pure bleach spilled onto skin can cause burns. To make a cleaning solution of 10 percent bleach, add 1 part bleach to 9 parts water. "Parts" just means any unit of measure; a part can be a capful or a bucketful.

Ethanol (drinking alcohol) is more expensive than bleach. Drinking ethanol can be used for cleaning, but less expensive ethanol can be purchased at chemical supply stores in many states. No license is needed. Drinking ethanol is very expensive because up to 40 percent of the retail price is government tax; chemical ethanol is not taxed. It is "denatured" (poisoned) so no one can drink it, but it can be used to clean needles. Ethanol does not harm metal but will eventually damage plastic.

A cleaning solution of ethanol should be at least 70 percent ethanol. This translates into "150 proof" for drinking alcohol. Using chemical ethanol, mix 7 parts of ethanol with 3 parts water to make a cleaning solution.

Isopropyl alcohol is rubbing alcohol. It can also be used to clean needles, although some epidemiological evidence suggests that it is not effective, perhaps due to improper technique. Isopropyl alcohol can be purchased at most drug stores and supermarkets. Examine the label to determine concentration. For some alcohols, a 70 percent concentration is not necessary. For additional information on the virus-killing activity of alcohols, see Chapter 19.

To clean the equipment, fill a container with the chosen cleaning solution. Stick the needle point into the solution and slowly draw the plunger back, filling the syringe. Keep the needle point below the surface of the liquid. Do not let air bubbles into the syringe. After filling the syringe, slowly push the plunger all the way to the bottom, expelling all the fluid from the syringe. Repeat this several times. Tap the syringe up and down its length to dislodge air bubbles.

After filling the needle and syringe a final time, disassemble the works and leave them soaking in the solution for at least 10 minutes. Preferably, let the equipment soak in alcohol until the next use.

Discard the cleaning solution after use. Discard any cleaning solutions left out overnight.

If the syringe contains blood, stronger mixtures of cleaning solution may be used.

If time is short, pour pure bleach into a glass, pump the bleach in and out of the syringe, then fill the glass with water, and pump some more. This procedure only takes a minute and reduces the risk of HIV transmission.

Before using the equipment, fill a glass with water and thoroughly flush the needle and syringe by pumping water in and out of the works. Change the water and rinse both the inside and outside of the equipment. Remove all smell of bleach.

Alternatively, the needles and syringe can be boiled for 10 minutes or more. This should kill HIV, but may not kill stronger bacterial agents.

Clean Technique. Before a needle is injected, the skin in the injection area should be cleaned with rubbing alcohol or 70 percent ethanol. If the area is visibly dirty, it should be washed with soap and water before wiping it with alcohol. After injection, IV drug users should immediately wipe off the needle with alcohol and clean it.

IV drug users should clean the works after use or before sharing. After injection, any blood spills should be cleaned with a bleach or alcohol solution. It is best to wear gloves when using bleach (grocery-store dishwashing gloves are fine). The cleaning solution should be left on the contaminated area for at least 10 minutes. Sponges and cleaning rags can be left overnight in cleaning solutions before being discarded or cleaned.

Needle Sharing. While some of the problems listed above are caused by unsterile needles contaminated by bacteria normally found in the environment, HIV transmission results from the sharing of needles. If no one shared needles or syringes, HIV transmission via IV drug use would cease.

No one should share hypodermic needles and syringes with another person; however, if this becomes necessary, the works should cleaned before the first person uses it, and before every use by another person. This should reduce the risk of HIV transmission.

Narcotics Anonymous (NA). NA is an organization created to help IV drug abusers and any person abusing drugs to kick their drug habits. NA is a volunteer organization created and run by addicts. Its only purpose is to help addicts kick the habit. All people are welcome, as long as they want to stop using drugs.

Modeled after Alcoholics Anonymous (AA), Narcotics Anonymous is very effective in helping addicts control and stop drug use. Members care about each other and demonstrate this caring by providing continual support.

NA does not attempt to solve the problems that underlie drug use. NA only attempts, quite successfully, to help the addict control his or her habit.

Drug abuse creates many problems. These problems can be cognitive, behavioral, physical, social, and economic. Many, though not all, of these problems are alleviated once drug use ends. Individuals through hard work and with adequate support, can construct a more healthy lifestyle.

Distribution of Needles. In Australia, Canada, France, Great Britain, the Netherlands, and Switzerland IV drug users are legally able to obtain sterile needles and syringes. Users may go to pharmacies or drug treatment centers and receive clean new needles and syringes, usually provided that they trade in their old "works."

Exchanging old works for new hopefully prevents careless addicts from leaving potentially infected needles lying about where children or other people may be stuck by them. The idea is to create a situation where the risk to both the addict and the public is as low as possible.

Amsterdam has the most aggressive needle exchange program. As a large international seaport, Amsterdam has become a center of the heroin trade and in recent years has had problems with a growing number of IV drug users, many of them foreigners. The government of the Netherlands has a strong commitment to all members of its society, and for years has had an aggressive drug treatment program for IV drug users. (Certain areas in the Netherlands tolerate the use of marijuana and hashish, although, contrary to popular belief, these drugs are not legal.) Using established treatment programs, Netherland authorities distributed 100,000 needles and syringes in an exchange program in 1985. At last record, only 2 percent (7/260) of the Netherland's AIDS cases are from IV drug use.

In England and Canada, the percentage of IV drug use-related AIDS cases hovers around 1 percent. In the United States, an estimated 16 to 25 percent of AIDS cases are related to IV drug use.

In Medical Settings

Blood Transfusions. The risk of contracting HIV from a blood transfusion is very small, so small that it is probably foolish to refuse blood transfusions in an emergency. (See Figure 21.)

While not all medical authorities agree with the procedure, more and more hospitals are offering *autologous transfusions*, meaning a patient is transfused with his or her own blood, donated before surgery. Only 1 in 10 hospitals allowed autologous transfusions in 1980.

Autologous transfusions also prevent other problems. Most negative reactions associated with transfusions are caused by foreign proteins (antigens) which the patient's body attacks.

Anyone planning elective surgery should consult his or her physician about autologous transfusions.

11. The Hope for a Vaccine

How a Vaccine Works

A vaccine is a substance which causes a person's body to produce antibodies against a disease without actually causing the disease. With viruses, antibodies are formed by T-cell recognition of viral protein coats or whatever antigenic (antibody-generating) substances the immune system is able to "see." The coats, or the proteins of the viral coats, are used to make a vaccine. Ideally, these antibodies are successful both in neutralizing the virus by latching onto it and in attracting cytotoxic (killer) cells to infected host cells.

To create a vaccine, technicians isolate and grow a large quantity of virus, then find a way to destroy its DNA or RNA center without destroying all of the protein coat. The viral coat, or crushed parts of it, are injected into a person's body. The person's immune system reacts to the presence of the viral proteins and creates antibodies to match them. The ability to make these antibodies remains with the person for years or, in some cases, for life.

If the vaccinated person later encounters a living form of the same virus and the virus gets into the bloodstream or lymphatic system, then antibody production begins immediately. Ideally, the antibodies will neutralize the virus before the virus can do any harm.

The Development of Vaccines

Substances which have potential use as vaccines are first tested *in vitro*. If there is a favorable result, the tests advance to small, inexpensive test animals, such as mice, guinea pigs, and rabbits. A promising candidate might be tried on monkeys, such as the rhesus monkey, but only the most promising substances get tested on chimpanzees.

Chimpanzees are very close to human beings in physical and metabolic functions. However, chimpanzees are an endangered species and difficult to breed in captivity. Consequently, they are very expensive and are saved for the most important experiments. At the time of this writing, there are only 1600 experimental chimpanzees in the United States, 300 of which are potentially set aside for AIDS research.

If a substance proves effective as a vaccine in chimpanzees, then it can be used in humans.

The Risks of Vaccines

Vaccines are not without risks. Sometimes all the DNA or RNA of the original virus is not destroyed, and strands, once injected into the body, are able to get into a host cell and begin replication. Then the vaccinated person gets the disease. This event is rare. Also, some people have negative reactions to vaccines, ranging from mild symptoms like a rash to severe ones like shock. Finally, vaccines may not work. The ability of the vaccine to generate antibodies varies from individual to individual, and some people do not generate anti-HIV antibodies. Vaccines proceed through a process of testing and development to prevent these problems, but even after they are in use with humans, there may be a period of adjustment before discovering the best methods of administration (e.g., intravenous versus intramuscular, one injection versus multiple injections over time, etc.).

Vaccines are risky for the first people who try them. The potential benefit must exceed the risk. Not all vaccines are given to everybody; some vaccines, such as the recently developed hepatitis B vaccine, are given only to certain high-risk groups, namely, health care workers who are often exposed to blood, and sexually active homosexual males. HIV, or course, presents a different situation. Unlike hepatitis B, HIV infection has no known cure.

With any potential HIV vaccine, members of high-risk groups will probably be the first vaccinated. While these groups greatly need the protection of a vaccine, there are some problems with being the initial test groups. First, there will be no guarantee that the antibodies produced by the vaccine will withstand a "challange" by HIV, that is, provide protection. It is unlikely that researchers will directly expose vaccine recipients to HIV. Ethically, a researcher cannot immunize a high-risk person and then encourage that person to engage in high-risk behavior to see if the vaccine works. Second, a person does not test positive for HIV as soon as he or she is exposed to it. If someone is vaccinated during this "window" period, after infection but before antibody development, the test results would be inaccurate. Seropositivity could result from either the infection or the vaccine.

Vaccines and HIV Mutation

Several problems present themselves in the development of an HIV vaccine. First, a 100-percent-effective vaccine has never been made for a retrovirus. With our current knowledge of biology and chemistry, it is theoretically possible to create such a vaccine, but in biology there are no guarantees. Second, different strains of HIV are now known to exist. That some of these strains have differing protein coats is demonstrated by the ELISA tests, tests made with HIV-1 as the antigen, which do not detect the HIV-2 virus.

In a similar fashion, the antibodies produced against one strain of virus may not work against another strain. Initially the hope was that a vaccine could be based on some antigenic part of the viral protein coat which remains the same for all strains of the virus. Such an antigenic site remains to be discovered. Otherwise, a vaccine would have to contain the antigens of all existing HIV strains to be effective against them all.

Even a vaccine containing antigens for all known HIV strains would be problematic because HIV mutates so quickly. Researchers now realize that HIV mutates at a rate 5 to 10 times faster than the influenza virus. The flu virus is an RNA virus for which a vaccine is available; however, a flu vaccine manufactured more than 2 to 3 years ago is no longer effective against the coming season's flu. The "antigenic drift," the change of the protein coats of the flu virus, has become too great for the antibodies of the old vaccine to remain effective. To put things in perspective, polio vaccines manufactured 30 years ago are still effective today; rabies vaccines manufactured 50 years ago are still effective.

There still remains the question of whether or not anti-HIV antibodies work against HIV. Antibodies are found in almost all HIV-infected people, but they do not seem to provide protection against HIV infection. Perhaps this lack of effective protection does not lie only in the antibodies. Perhaps some other undiagnosed problem exists which prevents the body from protecting itself.

Vaccine Strategies

Researchers are using a number of different approaches to vaccine development. The following is an overview of these approaches.

Attenuated Virus. One possible way to make a vaccine is to take the chosen virus and destroy the most important segments (genes) of its RNA or DNA content. A collection of these *attenuated* (shortened) viruses is then injected into the patient. The attenuated viruses should not be able to reproduce, but their whole protein coats should cause the development of effective antibodies against the whole virus.

An attenuated virus is not considered likely for HIV because there is always the risk that not all of HIV's RNA will be destroyed. It is possible that RNA fragments may remain in attenuated HIV viruses and that these fragments may hook up with promotors and enhancers (triggering genes) belonging to the host and become oncogenic (cancer-causing). Retroviruses also tend to recombine, and it is possible that RNA fragments might recombine to form a whole replicating strand. Finally, some studies suggest that the HIV envelope itself is cytopathic, causing the death of T-cells.

Killed Virus. Some scientists would argue that a virus cannot be killed, since it is not really alive. However, for a "killed" virus vaccine the RNA or DNA core is separated from the antigenic protein coat. This separation means that some of the antigens (proteins in the coat) may be lost and that antibodies produced in response to the vaccine may not be as effective against the complete protein coat. The cell-killing potential of the HIV envelope might also remain a problem with such a vaccine.

Subunit Vaccines. Subunit vaccines would be made from a small portion (subunit) of the virus's protein coat or a subunit of the molecules found on the envelope. The use of subunit vaccines would prevent any potential recombination which would reactivate an attenuated virus. Subunit vaccines would not contain any genetic material. However, a subunit of the protein coat may or may not be cytopathic to T-cells, and a subunit vaccine could fail to generate an adequate antibody response. The immune system may "see" a part less effectively than it sees a whole. One study using chimpanzees reveals that a single subunit vaccine may not be effective against HIV. Eight chimpanzees were injected with the purified proteins of the HIV envelope (gp 120). The chimpanzees manufactured antibodies in response to these protein subunits, but the antibodies did not prevent the chimpanzees from becoming infected.

Combinations of subunits may be needed for a vaccine to be effective. Theoretically, such combinations might be constructed into a rosette, a protein and lipid (fat) ball with HIV gene products chemically fixed to its surface. This type of structure is still theoretical.

Subunit vaccines have been the focus of most HIV vaccine strategies. Researchers are trying to create the subunits themselves, using genetic engineering techniques. In genetic engineering, scientists take the genes of one organism and implant them inside another. The genes of these experimental organisms are artificially "recombined." In attempting to create an AIDS vaccine, technicians remove the HIV genes responsible for creating the protein coat (*env*) and insert this HIV gene into the genes of another cell or virus. The resulting recombinant organism, when provided with nutrients and stimulated to grow, then turns into a factory, manufacturing relatively high quantities of the substance encoded in the implanted gene.

Scientists have inserted HIV genes into several types of cells, namely: (1) mammalian cells (cells of mammals); (2) yeast cells; (3) bacteria; (4) insect cells; and (5) the vaccinia virus. Researchers have had varying success with these techniques.

Mammalian cells have thus far shown the most promise. The gene proteins of HIV created by recombinant mammalian cells have generated anti-HIV antibodies in laboratory animals. An experiment on chimpanzees using purified recombinant *env* products did cause the creation of antibodies. However, when challenged with HIV, the antibodies did not prevent the infection of the chimpanzees, nor did they prevent the chimpanzees from getting ill. In another test using human blood, the mammalian-produced recombinant products did prevent HIV replication *in vitro*.

Antibodies created by the gene products of *recombinant bacteria* have also been created. These antibodies have been shown to produce anti-HIV antibodies in mice. Recombinant insect cells have also produced gene products which can stimulate the production of antibodies in laboratory animals. However, the gene products of bacteria and insect cells are not glycosylated (lack of certain sugar structures on their molecules). These sugars are evidently not necessary for antibody production, but the lack of them may affect the effectiveness of the antibody.

The *vaccinia virus* is a large virus often used by medical professionals and vaccine researchers. Since it is a large virus, a number of foreign genes can be spliced into its genetic material. Evidently, the French researcher in Africa who infected himself with a vaccine substance used a recombined vaccinia virus. One major advantage of the vaccinia virus is that it can be used alive. Thus a living, replicating source of HIV gene products might be introduced into the human body, providing an indefinite source of anti-HIV antibody production. A disadvantage of this virus is that it causes illness in some individuals. The gene products of this recombinant vaccinia virus reportedly stimulated the production of both anti-HIV antibodies and anti-HIV cytotoxic cells. These antibodies were not challenged by living HIV. After initial media acclaim, nothing more has been heard on this development.

Other experiments using recombinant vaccinia virus products (gp 41 and gp 120) with macaque monkeys have shown that these products do stimulate antibody production. Macaques, however, do not get AIDS; they get SAIDS, which is caused by another virus. Chimpanzees are the only animals who can be successfully infected and made ill by HIV.

Anti-Idiotype Antibodies. To create *anti-idiotype* antibodies, a virus protein is injected into an animal. The animal makes antibodies against the viral protein. These antibodies are then injected into another animal and this second animal makes anti-antibodies against the original antibodies. These anti-antibodies are called anti-idiotype antibodies. Anti-idiotype antibodies "look like" the proteins of the virus. (This process is similar to the way plaster of paris is used to make molds of a footprint. First the plaster is poured into an indentation in the dirt, making an inverse (opposite) mold. Then the inverse mold is filled with plaster of paris to make a "positive" image of the original footprint as it appeared pressed into the soil.)

Anti-idiotype antibodies, when injected into a person, should stimulate the production of antibodies which are also capable of latching onto real HIV. The anti-idiotype antibodies should be safe, since they contain no actual proteins or genetic material of the original virus. However, since they mimic the structure of the virus's protein, these anti-idiotypes may imitate the cytopathic effects of HIV.

Summary

Much testing and development of HIV vaccines remain to be done. During HIV infection, the body creates several types of anti-HIV antibodies directed against several HIV gene products. Currently, most vaccine efforts are focusing on the *env* gene product (gp 120), the protein of the viral coat, and its related antibodies. The effectiveness of antibodies directed against other HIV gene products needs to be examined. Combinations of the antibodies must also be examined.

Success in the laboratory or success in a limited number of animals or even humans is still a far cry from the development, large-scale manufacture, and distribution of a workable vaccine to the world's doctors. Estimates vary of the time before a workable vaccine will become available. Current estimates range from 4 to 15 years.

No one truly knows when, and if, HIV vaccine will be developed. It would not be wise to rely upon the development of a vaccine to solve the AIDS problem. Most likely, a vaccine will not help anyone who has already been exposed to HIV, and so people must protect themselves against exposure *now*.

12. Characteristics of the AIDS Epidemic

The size of the AIDS epidemic remains a mystery. No one knows how many people are infected with HIV, but information is now becoming available which sheds light on the size and shape of the AIDS epidemic. Presently in the United States and worldwide, HIV infection exists in pockets. Most HIV-infected people are found in urban centers. Strong regional differences exist in the percentage of population infected, the rates and risk of infection, and the types of people infected. When information is given concerning AIDS or the populations infected with AIDS, it may reflect a national average, or information gathered regionally.

History

Some time in the late 1970s, HIV was introduced into the homosexual male population of the United States. Around the same time, the first few batches of HIV-infected blood were collected for transfusions or for making coagulation factor for hemophiliacs.

Unfortunately, some of the first homosexual males to be infected were probably fast-laners, men who have sex frequently with anonymous partners. The first 50 AIDS patients studied were homosexual males who, on average, claimed more than 1100 sexual partners. Moreover, these men reported frequent anal intercourse, the most effective method of sexual transmission of HIV.

It was what we now call high-risk sexual activity that allowed HIV to establish its threshold. The *threshold* represents a percentage of the host population. At or above threshold, a disease is able to perpetuate itself in the population. If the disease does not achieve threshold, it does not successfully infect the "herd" and gradually dies out. For example, for measles to perpetuate itself in a city of 100,000 people, at any one time, 7000 people must be infected.

Unfortunately for humans, a second group of people who practiced another high-risk behavior, IV drug users, overlapped the homosexual male group. Some of the homosexual males who use IV drugs shared the needles with other people and transmitted HIV. Because they introduce HIV directly into the bloodstream, IV needles may be an even more effective method of transmitting AIDS than anal intercourse. The spread of HIV into the IV drug user population quickly increased the number of HIV-infected females, who were either IV drug users themselves, or sexual partners of male IV drug users. The female IV drug users and female sexual partners of male IV drug users are the primary sources of HIV-infected children.

Appearing around the same time as cases in the population of IV drug users were the AIDS cases due to blood transfusions and blood products in hemophiliacs and blood recipients. The infected female population was increased again by the cases among wives of hemophiliacs. The currently small heterosexual male and female HIV-infected population is growing to an unknown extent.

At the beginning of an epidemic, a germ spreads rapidly, transmitted very effectively by high-risk behaviors. As the epidemic progresses, almost everyone exhibiting those behaviors becomes infected. Depending on how large this group is, the germ may or may not achieve threshold.

Once the high-risk groups are infected, less efficient means of transmission become more important in increasing the size of the infected population. As the number of HIV-infected people grows, HIV transmission by low-risk behaviors becomes more likely. Therefore HIV transmission by contamination of the blood supply, by workplace accidents involving health care and dental workers, and by transmission via heterosexual activities will all increase.

Rate of Growth

In the initial stages of the AIDS epidemic, the doubling time of AIDS was 6 months. The *doubling time* is the time required for the number of cases to double. As the epidemic grew in size, the doubling time of the epidemic lengthened. As measured by the epidemic's doubling time, the rate of growth is slowing down. However, this slowing of doubling time does not mean that the epidemic is not still gaining momentum. Doubling of 5 to 10 AIDS cases or 100 to 200 is far different from doubling of 40,000 to 80,000 people, even though the doubling time is longer. The doubling time has slowed because HIV must rely on less effective means of transmission. The AIDS epidemic is still growing and at a dangerous rate, considering the mutability of the virus and current options of treatment.

A better measure of the epidemic is the annual number of AIDS cases reported. Thus far it keeps growing, but, at some point, the annual number will level off at equilibrium. *Equilibrium* is a state of being evenly balanced. At equilibrium, the annual number of AIDS cases stays approximately the same. For example, each year approximately 23,000 cases of hepatitis B are reported to the Centers for Disease Control (CDC). Hepatitis B has reached equilibrium at 23,000 new cases a year. Gonorrhea's equilibrium is almost 1 million new cases per year. A pathogen's equilibrium in its host population can be affected by a number of things. HIV is not considered to be as infectious as either of the pathogens which cause hepatitis B or gonorrhea, but the annual incidence has already climbed to 17,000.

Aids-Related Statistics

Statistics related to AIDS have an interesting ability to be warped out of realistic context. A common, particularly poor practice of twisting AIDS facts is the use of percentages rather than the use of absolute numbers. For example, between August, 1984, and August, 1985, the number of AIDS cases in males caused by heterosexual contact increased by 320 percent, while the number of cases caused in males by homosexual/bisexual contact increased by only 104 percent, making heterosexual contact the "fastest-growing area of AIDS transmission." In absolute numbers, a 320 percent increase meant that the number of male heterosexual cases increased from 5 to 21 cases. In comparison, the number of male homosexual/bisexual cases increased from 2200 to 4500. The same sort of statistical abuse has led to the report that a high percentage of minority female cases are due to contact with bisexual men. A high percentage of minority females contracted AIDS from bisexual partners compared to white females. As of Fall 1987, a total of 101 females, all races, had contracted AIDS that way.

Where the Numbers Come From

In the early years of the AIDS epidemic, the estimates of the extent of HIV infection were based on a study of 474 homosexual men who participated in a trial hepatitis B vaccine program in San Francisco. When their blood samples were reexamined, it was found that 1 percent of the men had antibodies to HIV in 1979. In the 1980 blood samples of this group, 23 percent had anti-HIV antibodies. By 1984, 67 percent of these men were seropositive. However, only 1 antibody carrier out of 28 (about 3 percent) in this group developed AIDS during this same time period.

In the Fall of 1985, a larger study of homosexual males was released. This study examined the histories of 6875 homosexual males who visited STD clinics in San Francisco between 1978 and 1984. Of the men carrying the antibody, 2 to 3 percent had developed AIDS with an additional 21 percent developing lymphadenopathy syndrome. The numbers suggested that only 2 to 3 percent of infected people developed AIDS. We know differently now.

These populations of homosexual men do not represent all homosexual men. These men were sexually active and attended an STD clinic. Not all homosexual men catch STDs, and not all homosexual men are sexually active. And this population of homosexual males does not represent the public as a whole.

At the present time, 36 percent of the HIV-infected men in this target group of San Francisco homosexuals have developed AIDS, and the likelihood is that the percentage will increase over time. While this reduces hope for those infected, it also lowers the estimate on the size of the unknown HIV-infected population. In 1987, the U.S. count of CDC-defined AIDS cases was 40,000. As one-third to one-half of all infected people, the total number of infected people would be estimated at approximately 80,000 to 120,000.

U.S. Military. Since October, 1985, the U.S. Department of Defense has screened individuals volunteering for military service for HIV. As of December, 1986, the Department of Defense had tested 789,578 people. Of these, 1186 tested positive by both an enzyme immunoassay similar to ELISA and by Western blot. Overall, 1.5 in 1000 people tested HIV positive. The prevalence varied according to sex, race, and ethnicity, and by home region of the applicant. (See Figure 21.)

What do these numbers mean? If volunteers entering the army reflect the general population of the United States, then in New England approximately 1 in 250 people who are 26 years of age or older are HIV-infected. In New Jersey, approximately 1 in 100 people 26 years of age or older are HIV-infected. By the same logic, 1 in 1700 people are HIV-infected in Montana.

The military studies are very important. The sample numbers are very large. However, military applicants do not represent the U.S. population as a whole. Volunteers are thought to underrepresent the three populations historically most affected by HIV infection, namely, IV drug users, homosexual males, and hemophiliacs. Hemophiliacs cannot pass medical standards for service. Since IV drug users and homosexuals must conceal these behaviors in order to remain in the service, it is *assumed* they are not as common in the military as in the general population.

Over the time span of these tests, there has been a slight decrease in the rate among white males (down 0.02 per 1000). The media reported this as a potential downturn in the epidemic. However, there has also been a growing awareness of the testing on the part of the public. This knowledge has probably reduced the volunteer rate of high-risk individuals.

American Red Cross. The Red Cross currently screens all donated blood for HIV. Their information provides a look at the testing procedure. One percent of all ELISA tests are positive on the first test. After Western blot testing, only 0.025 to 0.04 percent of blood donors are both ELISA and Western blot positive for HIV. These figures indicate a blood donor seroprevalence rate of HIV in the United States somewhere between 1 in 2500 people to 1 in 4000 people. Blood donors do not represent the general U.S. population. Members of high-risk groups are encouraged and constantly reminded not to donate blood.

CDC Hospital Surveillance Program. The Centers for Disease Control (CDC), working jointly with other federal agencies and local and state health departments, has created a small testing program. Anonymous blood samples from hospitals across the country are sent to CDC for testing. The hospitals have been selected in order to represent differing socioeconomic and demographic groups. Each hospital provides 300 specimens monthly, each marked with the patient's age, sex, and race. The source hospital is not revealed. Patients are not told their blood is selected, and CDC does not notify the patients of serpositivity. This program will provide CDC with 52,500 samples in the first year and is likely to be expanded.

Again, this testing program does not sample a population that represents the U.S. population. Sick people in hospitals are a special group.

Differences in AIDS Patients

Historically, AIDS has appeared primarily in special populations, namely, people practicing high-risk behaviors and their sex partners, and has centered in certain geographic locales.

Homosexual Males. Homosexual males are the predominant group in the AIDS epidemic. Most medical and social information available on AIDS and HIV stems from studies involving homosexual males. For the purpose of this book, a homosexual male is defined as a male who has sexual activity with another male, whether he engages in sex with females at the same time or at other times. According to a large poll of the U.S. population by Kinsey, about 4 percent of American males (2.5 million) are exclusively homosexual and 8 to 16 percent (5 to 10 million) have had homosexual experiences.

Figure 21: U.S. Military Screening Results

Listed here, by age group and region of residence, are the seroprevalence rates of HIV among civilian applicants for military service: October 1985—December 1986. These numbers represent "per 1000 tested." For example, 0.4 means that, out of 1000 people, 4 tenths of one person tested positive, or 1 person in 2500.

| Region | Age Group | | | |
	Between 17–20	Between 21–25	Greater than 26	All Ages
New England	0.4	1.0	3.8	0.9
Middle Atlantic	0.7	4.6	10.0	2.9
EN Central	0.4	1.8	1.9	0.9
WN Central	0.2	1.0	1.8	0.6
South Atlantic	0.9	3.4	5.4	2.1
ES Central	0.4	1.9	1.3	0.9
WS Central	0.6	2.7	3.0	1.6
Mountain	0.3	1.5	1.9	0.9
Pacific	0.8	1.5	4.0	1.5
US Territories	1.6	6.3	12.3	5.8
All Regions	0.6	2.5	4.1	1.5

In the beginning of the AIDS epidemic, the appearance of HIV infection in homosexual males was associated with multiple sexual partners or frequent receptive anal intercourse. Early statistical studies with these findings were conducted in San Francisco and New York City. However, later studies in Boston and Denmark did not show a clear-cut association between the number of sex partners and seropositivity. Currently, among the homosexual male populations of New York, San Francisco, and London, studies estimate 40 to 60 percent are HIV carriers. These associations only indicate how HIV has been transmitted historically. The future may bring changing patterns.

The symptoms of HIV infection are more clearly recognized in homosexual males than in any other group. Almost 50 percent of homosexual AIDS patients (CDC-defined) had oral symptoms of HIV infection: candidiasis, oral hairy leukoplakia, or herpes. Over 95 percent had lymphadenopathy of the head and neck. A large number of homosexual male AIDS patients have Kaposi's sarcoma as the first symptom of the disease, and Kaposi's sarcoma is generally very common in this group of AIDS patients. Some evidence exists now that cytomegalovirus, an infection common among some groups of homosexual males, is a cofactor of Kaposi's sarcoma.

Another problem common to AIDS patients of this group are lymphomas, cancers of the lymphatic system. An increasing amount of evidence suggests that these cancers are caused by abnormal B-cell proliferation. Lymphomas are frequently found in people who are not immunosuppressed by HIV. However, when HIV infection is present, the lymphomas are not restricted to the lymph nodes. Rather, they appear in the central nervous system, bone marrow, bowel, rectum, and skin.

Figure 22: Transmission Categories

Category	Description	Presence of Antibodies
Homosexual or Bisexual Males % of AIDS cases: **66%**	Includes any male who has one or more homosexual experiences in his life.	In high risk areas, an estimated 50% to 70% of homosexual males have antibodies to HIV. In low to intermediate risk areas, an estimated 10% to 50 % have antibodies to HIV.
Homosexual Male Intravenous (IV) Drug Users % of AIDS cases: **8%**	These individuals may have contracted AIDS either from high-risk sexual activity or from sharing intravenous needles.	No information available.
Heterosexual Intravenous (IV) Drug Users % of AIDS cases: **16%**	The majority of females with AIDS (49%) are IV drug users. Percentages of AIDS cases due to IV drug use are much lower in Canada and England where hypodermic needles may be legally purchased.	50% to 70% in high risk areas; 1% to 30% in low to intermediate risk areas.
Heterosexuals % of AIDS cases: **4%**	This is the only category where females outnumber males. A large percentage of female AIDS patients contracted it from male partners who were IV drug users. The percentage of heterosexuals is distorted because all foreigners with AIDS, such as Haitians, have been placed in this category. This group jumped from 1% to 4% of all AIDS cases when foreigners were taken out of the Undetermined category and placed in the Heterosexual category. While there are 1644 individuals in the category, 742 people (583 men, 160 women) who had "no other identified risk who were born in countries in which heterosexual transmission is believed to play a major role" (CDC definition). Another 902 persons (196 men, 706 women) had sex with persons with AIDS or at risk for AIDS. In summary, excluding foreigners, the percentage of heterosexual AIDS cases in U.S. citizens increased from 1% in 1985 to approximately 2% to date.	Varied. Reported 35% of women who were sexual partners of AIDS men. 25% to 70% of female sex partners contracted AIDS from their long term monogamous sex partners according to very small studies.

Hemophiliacs % of AIDS cases: **1%**	Received blood-clotting factors. Exposure should decrease with current safeguards and new technological developments.	Those receiving Factor VIII concentrate: 70% to 90%. Other coagulation therapies: 10% to 30%.
Transfusion Recipients % of AIDS cases: **2%**	Claimed no other known risk factors within five years of transfusion. Should decrease with current safeguards.	Unknown. Very rare.
Undetermined. % of AIDS cases: **3%**	Includes dead and never classified individuals; those who refused to supply information, those whose information is not yet available; and men who reported one heterosexual contact with a prostitute.	Seroprevalence studies of supposed low-risk populations showed ranges of 0.01% to 1% antibody presence.
Children: Under 13 years of age.	79% born to parents with/at risk for AIDS. 12% transfusions recipients. 5% hemophiliacs 4% no known risk factor.	Unknown. Very rare.

Approximately 42,000 adult cases and 600 pediatric cases were reported to the Centers for Disease Control (CDC) as of October 1987. Percentages given in this chart are cumulative for the whole of the AIDS epidemic. In adults, 93% are male; 7% female. In children, roughly 50/50 sex-wise. Estimated 10 to 15% cases not reported. Estimated 10% increase expected due to September 1987 redefinition of AIDS survelliance definition. Greatest majority of cases in individuals 20 to 49 years of age. Ages 30 to 39 contains 47% cumulative cases. Source: AIDS Weekly Survelliance Report, CDC, September 21, 1987.

In some urban areas, the U.S. homosexual male population is believed to have a germ pool containing a number of viruses and intestinal parasites that are not as common among heterosexuals. These persistent viruses may constantly activate the immune system in homosexual men. The new theory that HIV easily infects only activated cells suggests that homosexual males would be particularly susceptible to HIV infection. Many homosexual males have histories of previous STDs, for example.

Some homosexual males engage in sex with many partners and practice receptive anal intercourse. Both of these activities are statistically associated with HIV infection. AIDS is not caused by these activities; rather HIV is transmitted from one person to another. Many homosexual males report a reduction of these behaviors, and a drop in the reported rates of anal gonorrhea (both in the United States and in England) supports these statements. The incidence of anal gonorrhea is considered a good monitor of unprotected (without condoms) sexual activity in the homosexual male population.

IV Drug Users. An estimated 750,000 people inject illegal drugs into their bodies at least weekly. As the AIDS rate of growth leveled off in homosexual males, the rate of growth among IV drug users took prominence. During mid-1987, IV drug users were the fastest growing population of HIV-infected people.

Shooting up with an intravenous (IV) needle does not cause AIDS. HIV causes AIDS. However, IV drug users are at risk because many share needles with each other. Thus they share each other's blood and whatever lives inside the blood, like HIV, hepatitis B, and other common infections. With the exception of blood transfusions, needle sharing is probably the best way of transmitting HIV infection. Inserting a contaminated needle into one's arm bypasses most of the body's defenses and places HIV directly in the bloodstream. Also, the needle wounds draw macrophages directly to the area. The same trauma may place HIV directly into peripheral nerves.

Contrary to the popular belief that IV drug users are beyond all hope and do not care about their own health, IV drug users actively try to avoid HIV infection. The fear of AIDS has led to a hot black market in clean needles. Unfortunately, many needles sold as new on the streets are simply repackaged used needles. Heat-sealing machines, available at hardware stores, can reseal the plastic bags used in hypodermic needle packaging. The packaging on these resealed needles is imperfect and can be detected on close inspection.

IV drug users are a diverse population. In addition to the stereotypical junkies who must steal to support their habits, there exists a large number of weekend junkies, who are able to keep jobs and only shoot up at night and on weekends. For example, the professional group with the greatest percentage of IV drug use is physicians. Physicians are not at risk for AIDS from IV drug use because they have access to both clean hypodermic needles and pharmaceutically pure drugs.

The majority of HIV-infected IV drug users in the United States is located in New York and New Jersey. There is a heavy predominance of blacks among them. The high numbers in New York and New Jersey may reflect a greater degree of needle sharing among black IV drug users than among their white counterparts. Needle-sharing practices probably vary from region to region. Studies in England have proved this to be the case in England.

In various studies across the United States the seroprevalence of HIV among drug users ranges from 20 to 70 percent. These small studies do not represent all IV drug users, since most participants were attending drug treatment programs or clinics. Presumably, most addicts remain hidden. Laboratory testing for many standard ills is less reliable among the IV drug-using population. The great number of antigens and immune complexes presumably present in active IV drug users may or may not adversely affect HIV tests.

The symptoms of HIV infection in IV drug users differ from those found in homosexual males. IV drug users have a very low incidence of Kaposi's sarcoma, which suggests that homosexual males are exposed to some cofactor that promotes its development. IV drug users, as a whole, die sooner after diagnosis than homosexual males, except in New York City where homosexual males die sooner, according to one study. The higher mortality rate of IV drug users may result from a lack of adequate medical care, or reflect the damage done to the body by IV drug use, or may be due to factors yet unknown.

Tuberculosis (TB) is found in HIV-infected IV drug users more often than in homosexual males or in any other group in the United States. For members of the IV drug-using population, shortness of breath, pneumonia, tuberculosis, and oral thrush are all indicators of HIV infection, and medical evaluation should immediately be sought. IV drug users often need to be informed or reminded that they can receive treatment at local city hospitals.

The presence of tuberculosis in IV drug users may reflect social and economic status, rather than stem directly from HIV infection. Tuberculosis, a nonopportunistic disease, was a major killer in the United States in the relatively recent past. For the greater segment of the U.S. population, the rate of tuberculosis became negligible because of improved hygiene and the availability of effective drug therapy. However, pockets of tuberculosis remain in the United States and worldwide. A closer examination of TB-infected IV drug users may reveal a population which, due to social or economic reasons, has had no medical care or medical evaluation in many years, if ever.

IV drug users probably have activated immune systems. They are constantly exposed to foreign antigens from other people's blood and skin cells and from other environmental and blood-borne germs. The immune systems of IV drug users are also suppressed at times from malnutrition and the effects of their recreational drugs.

Women. Until 1986, women totaled only 7 percent of AIDS cases. Most were between 13 and 39 years of age, over half were black, and almost one-quarter were hispanic.

The majority of these females are IV drug users—52 percent. The second most common female risk group, 21 percent of the total, is the heterosexual sex partners of males belonging to a high-risk group, namely, male IV drug users, hemophiliacs, and transfusion recipients. In females who contracted HIV sexually, infection is strongly associated with long-term monogamous sexual activity with an infected male.

Some initial evidence indicates that HIV infection is more deadly in females than in males. Females die faster. Whether this is due to some physical difference between males and females, whether it reflects the socioeconomic factors of the disproportionate number of disadvantaged females with AIDS, or reflects a tendency in women to seek medical attention at a later stage of the disease is not known. Also, female medical complaints are taken less seriously by doctors than male medical complaints, a factor which could possibly be important considering the vague symptoms of HIV infection. The numbers for women are still small, and the statistical findings are not as certain.

HIV is definitely present in the U.S. female prostitute population. In Seattle, Washington, 5 out of 99 prostitutes tested positive for the anti-HIV antibody. In Miami, Florida, 10 out of 25 prostitutes reporting to an AIDS screening clinic tested positive to the antibody. Eight of these ten women were also IV drug users. The few studies of prostitutes available reveal that a small percentage are HIV-infected. A consistent finding is that most infected prostitutes are also IV drug users.

Prostitutes in Africa reflect a different pattern. In several small studies, seroprevalence rates range from 50 to 84 percent. Most of the studies were of prostitutes visiting STD clinics, and some of the sample sizes were very small. Few prostitutes were found to have any symptoms of AIDS besides swollen lymph nodes. IV drug use among African prostitutes is reportedly uncommon. Presumably, African prostitutes contracted AIDS through sexual activity. Other possibilities are that test accuracy is low or the tests are detecting antibodies or immune complexes for viruses other than HIV.

Heterosexuals. Most information on heterosexual HIV transmissions comes from the study of hemophiliacs and their wives and male IV drug users and their sexual partners. Consequently, HIV transmission from males to females is well documented. It has been repeatedly demonstrated that males can transmit HIV to females. Few cases of female-to-male transmission are documented, but they do exist. Presumably, males transmit sexually transmitted diseases to females more effectively than the reverse. Men outnumber women in all risk categories except in the heterosexual category where women outnumber men. In one sense, women are at a greater risk because more men have the virus than women.

Minorities. In the United States, a disproportionate number of AIDS cases are minorities, primarily blacks and hispanics. As of Fall 1987, 24 percent of all AIDS cases were black and 14 percent were hispanic, whereas these groups only compose 12 percent and 6 percent, respectively, of the U.S. population. (See Figure 22.)

Homosexual/bisexual males are the predominant group in all the racial groups mentioned. In both blacks and hispanics, IV drug users are the second largest group, accounting for 35 percent of AIDS cases in each group. In whites, IV drug users account for 5 percent. Together, blacks and hispanics account for 80 percent of all AIDS cases contracted by IV drug use.

The social and economic factors associated with IV drug use among minority populations are well known. However, these social and economic factors do not strongly affect the practice of homosexuality as evidenced by AIDS. Among homosexual males (who were not IV drug users), 74 percent were white, 15 percent were black, and 10 percent were hispanic as of September, 1986.

Strong racial prejudice exists among the U.S. homosexual population. In many U.S. cities, blacks are not allowed into white gay clubs. White homosexuals are, on the average, more educated and of a higher economic status than minority homosexuals; at least this is true for homosexuals with AIDS. While the white homosexual male population rapidly responded to the AIDS epidemic with money, organizations, and educational programs, the minorities were not, for the most part, a component of this effort. Thus, the slightly higher percentages of HIV-infected minority homosexuals may reflect a time lag in distribution of AIDS information and education to minority communities.

As evidenced by Figure 23, a disproportionate number of AIDS cases among blacks and hispanics are heterosexual individuals. A ballooning effect of the numbers here stem from two sources. First, a large number of these minority individuals are foreigners from countries "where heterosexual transmission is believed to play a major role," which are classified as minorities in the CDC classification system. Second, a significant number are female sex partners of male IV drug users.

Reports have suggested that minority women are at exceptionally high risk of catching AIDS from a bisexual male. Among women who are reported to have caught AIDS in this manner, 47 percent are white, 35 percent are black, and 14 percent are hispanic. In Fall 1987 a total of only 51 women had caught AIDS in this way. This group is too small for valid statistical analysis.

From 1981 to 1986, the ratios among minorities, relative to each other and to whites, have remained basically the same.

Minorities are not at a higher risk for HIV infection. A disproportionate number of IV drug users and prostitutes are members of ethnic minorities. Both social and economic factors account for this fact. All IV drug users and prostitutes are subgroups within their respective populations and are as isolated from other members of their minority groups as they are from society as a whole. Thus, as in the rest of society, individuals from minority groups who practice high-risk behaviors will quickly become infected, providing a threshold population that will eventually infect some of those at lower risk.

Most minority AIDS cases in the United States are located in New York, New Jersey, and Florida.

The discussion above relates to adults. Minority children account for the vast majority of pediatric AIDS cases. Black and hispanic children account for almost 80 percent of AIDS cases among children. Most of these children were born to mothers who were IV drug users or sex partners of IV drug users.

Hemophiliacs. Hemophilia is the medical term given to coagulation disorders of the blood. Coagulation is the drying up of blood to close wounds and form protective scabs. Hemophilia is inherited from one's mother and appears only in males. Females may carry the genes for hemophilia, but these genes have no effect on females.

Figure 23: Ethnic Breakdown — United States

	White	Black	Hispanic	Other/Unknown	TOTAL
Adult	61%	24%	14%	1%	100%
Child	21%	54%	24%	1%	100%

Adult				
Trans-mission Category	AIDS cases in **Whites**	AIDS cases in **Blacks**	AIDS cases in **Hispanics**	AIDS cases in **Other/Unknown**
Homosexual or Bisexual Males	80%	40%	49%	71%
Heterosexual IV Drug Users	5%	35%	35%	10%
Homosexual IV Drug Users	8%	7%	7%	5%
Heterosexuals	1%	11%	4%	2%
Hemophiliacs	1%	—	—	2%
Transfusion Recipients	3%	1%	1%	5%
Undetermined	2%	5%	4%	6%
Racial Totals:	≈100%	≈100%	≈100%	≈100%

Children				
Trans-mission Category	*AIDS cases in* **Whites**	*AIDS cases in* **Blacks**	*AIDS cases in* **Hispanics**	*AIDS cases in* **Other/Unknown**
Parent with/at risk of AIDS	46%	89%	82%	80%
Hemophiliacs	16%	2%	4%	20%
Transfusion Recipients	32%	6%	9%	—
Undetermined	6%	3%	4%	—
Racial Totals:	≈100%	≈100%	≈100%	≈100%

Notes: Other/Unknown includes Asian/Pacific Islanders and Native Americans including Alaskan Natives. The Black and Hispanic groups include foreigners, leading to a distortion of the heterosexual transmission category. The heterosexual category of these same ethnic groups also contain most of the females who contracted AIDS sexually from male IV drug users. Children are under 13 years of age.

Contrary to popular belief, hemophiliacs are not likely to bleed to death from small cuts. The problem hemophiliacs face is damage from internal bleeding into joints, muscles, or organs, leading to crippling and early death.

In the 1960s coagulation factors VIII (FVIII) and IX were discovered. Soon after their discovery, these coagulation proteins became available as commercial products, administered to hemophiliacs either at home or at treatment centers.

During the commercial manufacture of these clotting factors, the blood of 2000 to 25,000 people is pooled. In the course of a year's treatment, hemophiliacs are exposed to the clotting factors (and any viruses that may have slipped through) of 100,000 to 300,000 people. Precautions have always been taken to remove viruses and antigens from the clotting factors. After HIV came along, manufacturers began heat-treating clotting factor VIII, which generally kills the virus. Unfortunately, HIV transmission from heat-treated factor VIII (FVIII) has been reported. Untreated factor IX, required by fewer hemophiliacs, has also been found to transmit HIV, as has cryoprecipitate, a less pure form of clotting factor rich in FVIII.

Manufacturers have been researching additional purification methods. In Fall 1987, the use of monoclonal antibodies to manufacture a completely safe clotting factor was reported. Although the cost will be high, reports indicate that it will be possible for hemophiliacs to avoid HIV transmission.

Among hemophiliacs, the progression of HIV infection to clinical illness does not seem to occur at the same rate as it does in homosexual males and IV drug users. One theory suggests that some hemophiliacs were not infected with living HIV, but only received anti-HIV antibodies or disrupted portions of the HIV envelope. In some hemophiliacs, the presence of the anti-envelope antibody (anti-gp120) without the presence of the anti-core antibody (anti-gp41) might be cautiously interpreted as the transmission of noninfectious HIV envelope proteins only. Others suggest that these nonliving antigens act as a vaccine by inducing the body into creating antibodies without actually causing the disease. If this occurs, then the accidental vaccination might provide hemophiliacs with some protection against living HIV, should subsequent exposure occur.

Hemophiliacs share the immune stimulation that is a potential problem in IV drug users and homosexual males. Because coagulation factors are pooled from thousands of donors, hemophiliacs are exposed to a great number of foreign antigens or viruses. Also, blood transfusions are immunosuppressive.

Blood Transfusion Recipients. In the United States between 1977 to the beginning of 1986, approximately 24 million people received about 80 million units of blood by transfusion. As of October, 1986, 424 transfusion recipients had developed CDC-defined AIDS. Virtually all these cases stem from transfusions that took place months to years earlier, many preceding 1983.

In 1983, the American Red Cross and the U.S. Public Health Service established blood donor education programs, warning people at high risk for HIV infection not to donate blood or tissues or organs.

In 1985, the first year the ELISA test became available, 0.04 percent (4 in 10,000) of all U.S. blood donations were seropositive for HIV. Assuming that each seropositive blood unit was transfused into a different recipient and assuming that all seropositive units transmitted infection, then 7200 individuals were inoculated with HIV by transfusions in 1984. Extending this back to 1981, up to 12,000 individuals acquired transfusion-associated HIV infection.

Routine tests for HIV infection are not a recommended priority for all blood transfusion recipients because the risk is low. The risk of contracting HIV by transfusion varies by region; it is highest in regions where HIV is most common. Multiply-transfused individuals are at a higher risk than individuals receiving only a few units of blood.

HIV is known to have a long incubation period. Blood transfusion recipients are among the few AIDS patients for which a date of inoculation is known. Generally, the course of the disease develops more rapidly after diagnosis in blood-transfusion recipients than it does in other risk groups. Presumably, this is because high concentrations of HIV are placed directly into the bloodstream. The onset of transfusion-associated AIDS has varied from 4 to 84 months after transfusion.

Africans. Since Central Africa is in the tropics, certain tropical opportunistic diseases are found in African AIDS patients that do not occur as frequently in U.S. or European AIDS patients.

Most African AIDS patients are of reproductive age with men averaging in their thirties and women in their twenties, who live in urban centers, who are members of the upper social class, and who report themselves to be heterosexuals with many sexual partners.

In the tropics, cryptococcal infections such as sepsis and meningitis; herpes infections of the mucous membranes, histoplasmosis (also found in Europe, but not in the United States), and cytomegalovirus infections of the eye, chorioretinitis, are found more frequently than in temperate zones. Tuberculosis, both localized and spread throughout the body, is more common among African AIDS patients. Oral and throat candidiasis are common among African AIDS patients, as is severe and persistent diarrhea, leading to more severe weight loss than is normally seen in U.S. AIDS patients. African AIDS patients tend to have pimply and itchy rashes at some point in the infection. Female AIDS patients frequently stop menstruating.

Kaposi's sarcoma and *Pneumocystis carinii* pneumonia are less frequently found in African patients than in U.S. and European patients.

The African information is rather limited. A number of theories suggest why AIDS apparently has spread so quickly among heterosexuals in Africa. First, it is likely that all tropical Africans are more frequently in an immune-activated state than are Europeans and temperate-zone Americans.

The tropics have a higher gradient of life than the earth's temperate zones, meaning there are more types of animals, plants, and microorganisms per square mile than in the temperate zones. Thus, theoretically, people living in the tropics are exposed to more diseases in their lifetimes than people in temperate zones. Their immune systems may be constantly challenged and in activated states.

A number of other possible explanations for the high rates have been suggested. As in most areas of the Third World, Africa does not have large medical industries. Reportedly, many hospitals and health centers reuse hypodermic needles. Reuse of improperly sterilized needles has been documented as a cause of polio in Third World medical settings.

Hypodermic needles in Africa are also used by traditional healers who think the instrument, not the medicine, has healing power. These healers inject one patient after another with these cherished needles. However, it seems unlikely that the educated members of the upper social classes, the population in which most AIDS cases are reported, frequent witch doctors.

Another theory suggests that medical needles are the avenue of HIV transmission in Africa. Most African AIDS patients and many other AIDS patients worldwide have histories of sexually transmitted diseases. In fact, many individuals tested in Africa were recruited from STD clinics. In this theory, improperly sterilized needles used at clinics are passing HIV from one patient to another. If this is true, then HIV was not initially transmitted by sex in Africa. Rather, sexually active individuals catch an STD, and then are infected with AIDS at their STD clinic.

Blood transfusions are another suspected avenue for HIV transmission.

Blood transfusions are more common in certain parts of Africa than in the United States. Blood transfusions are reportedly used to treat malaria and other chronic diseases, often in the absence of other medical treatment.

Other methods of transmission which have been suggested are tribal tattooing and scarification rituals, male circumcision, and female clitorectomies. Blood-letting instruments may infect an entire group of people. However, clitorectomy is reportedly not found in the areas of Africa presently infected with AIDS and the urban elite with AIDS may no longer practice these traditional rituals.

The sex ratio of AIDS cases in Africa is reported as 1 to 1 (1:1). In most studies, such statistics are "adjusted" for age differences. However, there seems to be a male predominance, after unadjusting the raw numbers for age differences.

It is difficult to estimate the extent of HIV infection in Africa. Zaire focused attention on its cases when, in 1983, it invited scientists to perform seroprevalence studies. It is unfortunate for Zaire that misleading information was extrapolated from these biased samples. The estimated incidence of HIV infection in Kinshara, Zaire, is roughly equal to the incidence of HIV infection in the United States.

Haitians. Initially, Haitians were classified as a separate high-risk group, just as homosexuals and IV drug users are considered to be high-risk groups. The presence of AIDS in Haitians was considered a mystery, whereas the AIDS in Africa was considered a sign of African origin. Haitians are no longer classified as a high-risk group, since it is now recognized that AIDS is transmitted in Haitians by the usual high-risk characteristics of homosexuality and perhaps prostitution, drug abuse, and blood transfusions.

Of those questioned, almost all Haitian AIDS patients in the United States denied homosexuality, bisexuality, or IV drug abuse. Many reported promiscuity, and males reported repeat encounters with prostitutes. Conversely, AIDS patients in Haiti reported a high incidence of bisexuality. Small studies on the general Haitian population in New York City suggest that HIV seroprevalence is low.

In the years preceding the AIDS epidemic, Haiti was a popular vacation spot for homosexuals from the United States. American gay publications carried advertisements of sex clubs and services in Haiti.

Concerning HIV transmission, Haiti has many of the same possible factors as Africa does, namely, unsanitary medical and traditional-healer use of needles, common blood transfusions, and tropical parasites. In addition, it has been suggested that certain voodoo rituals may spread AIDS. In voodoo ceremonies, the brains and blood of dead people are handled by voodoo priests. These brains and blood are mixed into a potion which the people attending the ceremonies drink. Whether these activities could transmit AIDS is not known. The consensus is that HIV could not survive the stomach's acids. No association between these activities and HIV infection has been found in studies.

Since Haiti is in the tropics, certain tropical opportunistic diseases are found in Haitian AIDS patients more commonly than in U.S. AIDS patients. Tuberculosis and central nervous system toxoplasmosis are common, as is infection by salmonella bacteria, a common agent of food poisoning. Kaposi's sarcoma and *Pnuemocystis carinii* pneumonia occur less frequently in Haitians than in North Americans. Oral and throat candidiasis is common among Haitian AIDS patients as are frequent gastrointestinal problems and pimply rashes.

13. The Question of Origin

The origin of AIDS, or rather the Human Immunodeficiency Virus (HIV), remains a mystery. As the gradual understanding of AIDS epidemiology grows, numerous theories regarding the origin of AIDS will develop. Already, a large constellation of AIDS-related facts exists, and these facts can be selectively assembled to illustrate any number of scenarios. However, with the information at hand, any origin theory resembles a connect-the-dots picture with no numbers. The theorist looks at the dots and connects them as he or she sees fit.

True to human nature, the various theories of the origin of AIDS differ according to the geographical location of the theorist. In the United States the popular belief is that AIDS comes from Africa. A popular belief among Europeans is that AIDS comes from the United States. In Africa, Europeans are thought to have brought the disease.

Little scientific inquiry into the origin of AIDS has been conducted. A common comment is that the origin is not important—only finding a cure is. However, in the modern world, where a disease can climb on an airplane and be across the world in half a day, knowing the origin of AIDS may be very important. The lessons learned from AIDS may save a few lives—next time!

African Origin Theory

Zaire is popularly thought to be the geographic origin of AIDS in Africa. Zaire was the first African nation to invite researchers to study AIDS and received much bad press for their efforts. Consequently, for a period of time Zaire did not report AIDS cases to the World Health Organization.

Zaire used to be called the Belgian Congo, and was once a colony of Belgium. Zaire still has economic and educational ties to Belgium, and educated Zairians, like most Belgians, speak French.

The first Africans reported to have AIDS were Zairians, diagnosed in Belgium where they lived. These first African individuals were self-proclaimed heterosexuals who were highly sexually active, well-educated, upper-class men, and their wives and children. Reports of these "African" AIDS cases filtered through the medical literature until 1983 when a group of researchers was invited to Zaire. These researchers found 38 cases of AIDS within a matter of weeks. No blood test was available in 1983, so these AIDS cases were diagnosed on the basis of clinical symptoms detected visually and by collection of medical histories. Based on these 38 cases, the researchers suggested that the AIDS rate in Zaire was 170 cases per 1 million people per year—a very high rate. Extrapolating further, it was predicted that millions of Africans would die over the next few years.

The ELISA test brought seroprevalence studies to Africa. From a variety of rather small studies came an avalanche of media reports. In various studies the seropositivity of African populations ranged from 2 to 98 percent. Unfortunately, these studies were often flawed by poor technique, and the results were distorted by the media. For example, in Zaire's capital city, 13 out of 26 female prostitutes tested seropositive. These individuals were "selected" from walk-in STD clinics and were not necessarily representative of African women, nor even of Zairian prostitutes. Nonetheless, in some media reports at that time, half of African prostitutes were said to have AIDS.

Meanwhile, humans were not the only organisms whose blood was being tested. Reports soon followed that the African Green monkey harbored the "AIDS virus," or a virus which was the link between humans and animals. This virus, "the missing link," was not HIV but SIVagm. SIVagm (Simian Immunodeficiency Virus in the African Green monkey) is not closely related to HIV, but to HIV-2 (HTLV-IV), which does not cause AIDS. More current evidence suggests that SIVagm migrated from humans to the monkeys.

Continued blood testing revealed some odd patterns of seropositivity. In cities, seropositive people tended to be upper-class, educated, and of the urban elite—the men in their thirties, women in their twenties. Additional random tests found HIV seropositivity to be high in several rural populations. Such testing included stored blood taken from a rural population in 1973. In the rural populations, HIV seropositivity was high in children, and generally became higher with age. Little or no disease was reported in these rural populations.

With this set of facts, an African-origin scenario can be constructed, which goes as follows: With the discovery of the supposed "AIDS virus" in African monkeys, the monkeys were assumed to be the original HIV reservoir, or the reservoir of HIV's ancestors. Monkeys can transmit disease to humans, as evidenced by *herpes simiae*, herpes virus. According to this theory, monkeys transmitted HIV to rural humans, the only humans they encounter. Presumably, most of the rural population becomes infected before adulthood. Since no AIDS or AIDS-like disease develops in these populations, it seems possible that HIV, if contracted during childhood, is not fatal; in fact, it does not cause disease at all. Thus, individuals surviving to adulthood are granted antibody-based immunity. A parallel situation exists with infectious mononucleosis, also known in the United States as the "kissing disease" and the "sleeping disease," caused by the Epstein-Barr virus.

By most estimates, the majority of individuals in the United States and Europe are exposed to the Epstein-Barr virus in childhood. (See Figure 10.) Minor clinical symptoms, or none at all, present themselves if infection occurs before 8 or 10 years of age. The individual creates protective antibodies. An older adolescent or young adult who, never previously infected, is exposed to the Epstein-Barr virus will probably display serious clinical symptoms, namely, mononucleosis.

The suggested shift of equilibrium causing the AIDS epidemic was the influx of rural people into the cities, caused by the social upheaval of westernization. Thus symptomless rural carriers were suddenly infecting nonimmune urban adults. One suggestion is that many rural females became prostitutes. No transmission link between Zaire and the United States or Haiti has been suggested that withstands examination.

New information has shed some light on this scenario. The monkey virus has been examined more closely and has been differentiated from HIV. Also, the accuracy of the ELISA tests is being questioned. There is a high correlation between a person having anti-malaria antibodies and testing positive for the antibodies to HIV, HTLV-I, and HTLV-II. This information can be intepreted in different ways: (1) anti-malaria antibodies or immune complexes "fool" the AIDS test, and (2) some other virus, pathogen, or condition which causes a positive reaction is present.

Some South American studies suggest that false-positives occur, for unknown reasons, in tropically based populations. In one study Venezuelan patients with acute malaria had high seropositivity rates, but no known risk factors and no signs of immunosuppression. In another study 3 to 13 percent of healthy aboriginal Amazonian Indians tested seropositive for HIV. Again, the subjects exhibited no disease, no risk factors, and virtually no contact with the outside world.

Unfortunately, the situation of AIDS in Africa is likely to remain unclear for the next few years, given the scarcity of information offered by existing studies, the varied reporting abilities of the various nations or regions, and the slow nature of HIV infection.

In Africa there is a disease called "slim disease." It is a wasting disease, meaning that ill individuals lose weight drastically, and this wasting leads to death. Since wasting is also a major factor in AIDS, it was inevitable that slim disease would be linked to AIDS. The U.S. popular media and some scientific journals have concluded that slim disease is AIDS. Unfortunately, very little scientific literature discusses or describes slim disease or compares slim disease to AIDS. Existing literature comparing the two diseases is not based on observations of patients. Rather, conclusions that slim disease is AIDS are based on literature reviews, that is, studies of case reports of respective patients. Death or morbidity due to weight loss from diarrhea can be caused by HIV infection or any number of parasites. Reports coming from Central Africa now indicate that wasting seems to be the predominant characteristic of AIDS in Africa, rather than opportunistic infections. It is possible that slim disease is AIDS because AIDS manifests itself differently in Africa. It is also possible that slim disease exists apart from AIDS and mistakenly is diagnosed as AIDS.

Haitian Origin Theory

When the presence of AIDS was discovered in Haitians who had immigrated to the United States, Haiti was cited as a possible site of the origin of AIDS. Alternatively, it was cited as a stepping-stone for AIDS as it traveled from Africa to the United States. This theory is losing credibility now that AIDS patients in Haiti are admitting to bisexual behavior, and with the recognition that Haiti hosted a number of homosexual sex clubs which were advertised internationally.

U.S. Origin Theories

As of 1985 the United States had 80 percent of the world's reported AIDS cases, according to the World Health Organization. However, a number of problems

Figure 24: The Global Situation

Continent	Number of reported AIDS Cases[1]
Americas	40,567
Europe	5,727
Africa	4,570
Oceania	521
Asia	150
Total	51,535

Country	Number of Reported Aids Cases[2]	Population[3]	Estimated AIDS cases per million
French Guiana	58	73,022	794
Haiti	851	5,272,000	161
U.S.A.	35,769	231,106,727	155
Congo	250	2,000,000	125
Rwanda	750	6,030,000	124
Trinidad & Tobago	134	1,176,100	114
Uganda	1138	12,636,179	90
Cent. African Republic	202	2,630,000	77
Burundi	285	4,480,000	64
Tanzania	1130	21,730,000	52
Canada	1000	25,358,500	39
Switzerland	227	6,445,900	35
Australia	481	15,751,510	31
France	1617	54,832,000	29
Denmark	150	5,116,975	29
Belgium	230	9,863,374	23
Dominican Republic	127	2,655,000	20
Gambia	14	695,886	20
Netherlands	260	14,453,833	18
W. Germany	1036	61,035,000	17
Brazil	1695	119,098,992	14
Kenya	286	20,000,000	14
U.K.	750	55,776,422	13
Sweden	110	8,342,621	13
Italy	664	57,128,000	12
New Zealand	45	3,307,837	12
Ivory Coast	118	10,056,000	12

Figure 24: The Global Situation (Continued)

Country	Number of Reported AIDS Cases[2]	Population[3]	Estimated AIDS cases per million
Ghana	145	12,205,514	12
Austria	72	7,551,800	10
Zaire	335	32,100,000	10
Spain	357	38,818,355	9
Israel	38	4,260,000	9
Mexico	407	78,800,000	5

Reported cases match Surveillance Definition of World Health Organization (WHO) which is virtually identical to the CDC Surveillance Definition, since CDC collaborated in its creation. Reported cases does not mean ALL cases. Reporting may vary from country to country, perhaps affected by economics and politics. Some countries do not report. Most countries having reported rates of greater than 12 cases per million are listed.

[1] Total number of AIDS cases reported to World Health Organization (WHO) as of June 1, 1987.

[2] Total numbers of cases reported to WHO, dates of reporting range from March 1987 to June 1987.

[3] Populations, circa 1979, are from census or estimates.

exist when studying *reported* cases. A popular belief is that there are more AIDS cases in Africa than are being reported, due to the lack of large medical infrastructures. Presumably most African AIDS patients belong to the upper social classes, who have access to the medical facilities that do exist. Based on limited observation, although a high percentage of rural individuals test seropositive for HIV, few have clinical signs of disease. However, the possibility that many unrecorded cases of AIDS exist in Africa must be considered.

The reports from the Soviet Union and the Soviet satellite countries have also been questioned. All these countries report extremely few AIDS cases. One possibility cited is that the Soviet Union and its allies are simply not reporting accurately, and that many more AIDS cases exist and they are hiding them. Another possibility is that the Soviet bloc has few AIDS cases because it is closed to Western travelers. Wherever AIDS originated, there is little doubt that internationally mobile homosexual males were instrumental in its spread throughout the free world. Since tourist travel to the Soviet bloc is restricted, these individuals had limited access to those countries. It is suggested that if Africa were the place of origin of AIDS, then the Soviet Union would have a higher incidence of AIDS, since the Soviet Union has strong trade links, which include exchanges of personnel, with many African states, and many African students attend Soviet universities.

Natural Origin. Possibly HIV has existed quietly for a number of years, and some recent event changed its equilibrium in the human host population. Or,

HIV might be the mutant of some other obscure virus which has been lingering at the fringes of human host societies.

Immunodeficiency is not medically unknown. Infants are sometimes born immunologically incompetent; immunodeficiency in these instances seems to be unrelated to HIV. A recent review of medical literature revealed 28 cases of Kaposi's sarcoma in the United States and Europe between 1902 and 1966. The individuals all had opportunistic infections (one had disseminated tuberculosis, rather rare except in AIDS cases), and all died within 3 years. These symptoms are similar to those of AIDS. The researchers suggest that HIV could be endemic (naturally occurring below troublesome epidemic rates) and that recent social and cultural changes increased its prevalence in the populations.

A similar development occurred with hepatitis B. Although hepatitis B has been a recognized problem for decades, it was endemic until the 1970s when its prevalence rapidly increased and it became epidemic among homosexual males and IV drug users.

Laboratory Origin. The scientific literature of England and Europe discusses the possibility of HIV being a man-made virus; scientific literature in the United States does not address this theory.

East German microbiologists suggest that HIV is a biological weapon, and conclude that HIV was created through genetic engineering. This is technically possible.

The U.S. military sponsors diverse biological research for both medical and weapons applications. A large proportion of this biological research is classified and, unlike most other scientific and medical research sponsored by other branches of the government, it goes unreported in the network of scientific literature.

On the other hand, HIV seems like a poor weapon: too difficult to transmit, too slow for battlefield use, even too slow to eliminate an enemy population, unless this population's main activities are sex, IV drug use, or blood-brother rituals. Finding a testing ground for HIV would also prove difficult, owing to its long incubation time and its reluctance to infect nonhuman primates. In order for HIV to be proved effective as a weapon, someone would have had to inoculate humans and follow their progress for many years.

If HIV did have a laboratory origin, an accidental escape would seem more likely than intentional inoculation. For example, visna virus, responsible for progressive neuropathy in sheep and, like HIV, a lentivirus, has been grown in human cell cultures since 1973 when it was cultured in human brain cells. This process is simply a reversal of what scientists usually do, that is, grow human pathogens in experimental animals.

Several studies indicate that animal viruses grown in human cells become more "human-tropic" over time. This means the cultured population of the virus, after several generations, consists primarily of individuals having the genetic and antigenic traits that best fit the environment of the human cells. While becoming human-tropic, the virus lessens its ability to infect the former animal host. Mutation provides the diversity; natural selection (the environment) decides which individuals survive. An equilibrium of diverse individuals exists all the time, their relative ratios varying according to environment.

The current library of HIV nucleotide sequences does not suggest any such link between HIV and any known laboratory lentivirus. Of all the viruses in the world, very few can live inside humans; the environment inside humans is hostile to most living things. However, genetic engineering and laboratory experimentation may be actually increasing the rate of genetic alteration in microorganisms, creating changes which occur rapidly, rather than the slow, incremental changes found in nature.

Vaccines

The recently created hepatitis B vaccine has been suggested as the vehicle for HIV entry into the United States from Africa or Haiti. Vaccines often contain human serum, the fluid portion of the blood. Serum is imported from the Caribbean and South Africa for use in pharmaceutical products. In the late 1970s, hundreds of homosexual males in San Francisco and New York City were injected with hepatitis B vaccine as part of human vaccine trials. Soon afterward, AIDS began to spread rapidly in the homosexual male populations of these cities. However, studies performed by the Centers for Disease Control, among others, indicate no statistical correlation between being a recipient of the hepatitis B vaccine and being HIV-infected. Also, reportedly, many health care workers also received hepatitis B vaccine injections and no epidemic development of AIDS in this population has been noted.

Later studies attempted to find evidence of HIV in hepatitis B vaccine preparations. No evidence of HIV antigens or HIV genetic material were found in the tested batches.

In another theory, the smallpox vaccine is suggested as the cause of AIDS. The smallpox vaccine contains the vaccinia virus which is known to trigger other viruses into action. In a campaign to eradicate smallpox, many Africans were vaccinated. It is suggested that the HIV virus was always present in African populations due to monkey bites and that the vaccinia virus triggered widespread AIDS. In addition, a large Haitian work force was present in Central Africa at that time, which could explain the transference of AIDS from Africa to Haiti. An argument against this theory is the lack of AIDS in children in Africa who have been vaccinated. Also, the monkey now seems an unlikely reservoir for HIV.

The United States–Europe–Africa Connection

Some unknown bridge has allowed HIV to span the thousands of miles separating the United States, Europe, and Africa. Europe and the United States are strongly linked by trade and tourism. The link between the United States and Central Africa is less distinct, although there is trade between Zaire and the United States. The HIV-1 isolates found in Central Africa are closely related to the HIV-1 isolates found in the United States and Europe, so presumably a connection does exist. Further research is needed on this point.

The recognition of AIDS in Africans, Haitians, and urban North Americans occurred roughly at the same time. Some scientists speculate that if HIV was introduced at the same time into Haiti, Zaire, and the United States, it would spread faster in the developing nations. The major reasons suggested are (1) the greater use of nonsterile hypodermic needles and syringes, (2) different sexual behaviors, and (3) frequent use of blood transfusions used to treat malaria and other parasitic and chronic diseases. Others argue the opposite, that transmission would happen faster in the United States, with its large populations of homosexual males and IV drug users.

The puzzling thing about AIDS is that it appeared suddenly, seemingly out of nowhere. Biology is a continuum of organisms generally traceable to some relative. A human and a virus must have ancestors; neither can spring fully formed out of thin air. Close examination of blood and serum products exported to and from the Third World might still reveal some vehicle used by HIV either to enter or leave the United States.

14. AIDS Education

Education works. Tuberculosis was largely defeated by public education efforts earlier this century. Education has also proved effective in reducing smoking behaviors in childhood and adolescence.

Unfortunately, there are large gaps in the area of health-related educational efforts. Our "modern" society, with all its scientific advances and social freedoms, still bears the legacy of the Victorian era.

If we repeat the mistakes of our cultural forefathers, we will force sex and any talk of sex back into the forbidden, and ignorance will strengthen its hold on our minds.

Some basic facts and principles related to health education are offered here.

Goals

Health education usually has several goals: (1) increasing knowledge, (2) changing attitudes, and (3) changing behavior. All three educational aims should be addressed. Ideally, any educational program should include a means of self-evaluation, measuring before and after effects.

Audiences. Four general audiences need education concerning AIDS: (1) the general public, (2) health care workers, (3) people engaging in high-risk activities, and (4) HIV-infected people. Each group has special needs.

Many subgroups exist within these four groups. Whatever the audience, the instructor must consider the audience's communication skills, values, and lifestyles. Instructors should try to accept the behaviors practiced by students without judgment or punitive reaction. With nonhealthy behaviors, initial acceptance establishes a foundation from which both teacher and pupil can work— one step at a time.

Content. All groups need basic information on HIV transmission patterns, epidemiology of HIV, AIDS prevention, and nonjudgmental, accurate information concerning homosexuality, drug abuse, death, and dying. Educators should cover all the issues and then highlight, review, or reinforce the group-specific issues. Questions should be encouraged.

The Problem. Most sex and drug education is punitive, promoting the idea that people who engage in sexual behavior or drug use are bad people, and that bad things should and do happen to them. In truth, every individual's personality contains both good and bad aspects, and most individuals engage in bad, or unhealthy, behaviors from time to time. Behavioral problems are a matter of degree. For one reason or another, some people tend to behavioral extremes. In theory, these people are using bad techniques to cope with stress or problems because they have had no opportunity to learn the good techniques.

There is obviously a role for positive, productive sexuality. Methods of dealing with one's own sexuality, strategies for engaging in healthful sex, and the ability to negotiate healthy sexual activities with one's partner, are all skills that individuals need to learn.

Unfortunately, the science of sex and the technology of sex education lag centuries behind other medical, scientific, and technological developments. Few empirical studies have measured the effectiveness of sex education. In these few, however, there have been positive results.

Children

In a controlled study, children exposed to health education demonstrated increased knowledge, healthier attitudes, better health skills, and better health practices, in regard to personal hygiene and cigarette smoking.

A study in an inner-city setting showed significant gains in knowledge for youngsters of both high- and low-income brackets regarding health-related behaviors. Education does work, an idea proved by notable lifestyle changes in smoking, exercise, and diet behaviors.

The Basics. Children need to know (1) the biological facts of reproduction, (2) the concept of sexually transmitted diseases, and (3) the very basic facts of AIDS. The best time to explain the biology of human reproduction to a child is before bodily changes of pubescence introduce teenage insecurity.

Initial sex education is biologically oriented, and thus it can be described as "the science of life" or "understanding our bodies." What children need to know is the function of the sexual organs, how sexual intercourse occurs, what menstruation is, how eggs are fertilized, how a fetus grows, and how a baby is born. Concepts of mating, parenting, and family creation should also be included.

Children also need to know that sexually transmitted diseases (STDs) exist. Children need not be confronted by medical terms. The concept of disease transmission is a simple one, presented as basic hygiene. (Wash your hands before dinner to kill the germs.) Children need to understand that by kissing, a person can catch the flu; by engaging in sexual intercourse, a person can catch something like a flu, only more serious.

Regarding AIDS, children need to know the basics: that AIDS is caused by a germ; that a person can catch AIDS from sexual activities; from blood transfusions, although this is unlikely; and from sharing hypodermic needles. They should know that AIDS can kill people, so that they understand how serious it is. The facts of IV drug use may need to be discussed, hopefully nonpunitively and with compassion for the afflicted.

Resistance Skills. It seems that children can learn and develop skills which aid them in resisting persuasion. Resistance is more than saying no. Under consistent pressure almost every individual eventually changes the no to yes. Additional strategies are required.

In situations involving peer pressure, several strategies are generally used. One method of resisting pressure is to find an *ally,* a friend. Two or more people can withstand pressure better than one; they can reinforce one another and perhaps form stronger friendships.

Avoidance is another way of offsetting pressure, perhaps physical avoidance of the place or situation in which pressure exists, or simple avoidance of the stressful subject by being quick to change the topic of conversation.

A person's *value* to a peer group may also offset group pressure. A person of value is less likely to be pressured to conform. This value can be based on personality, achievements, knowledge, or any number of things.

The development of resistance skills is an area in need of additional research.

Teachers. An embarrassed teacher is a problem. In essence, we need to instill new knowledge and new abilities into today's children, and we are doing it with tools forged centuries ago in fear and ignorance. If teachers cannot say penis and vagina without flinching, then sex education specialists may be needed. In one small study the classes which learned the most were taught by teachers who were interested in teaching sex education.

Parents' Role. Parents need to be aware that sex education is part of the school curriculum and be prepared for the blunt and sometimes tactless questions that only a child can ask. Ideally, parents are comfortable with their sexuality and with talking about sex, and can answer the child's questions without embarrassment, and without burdening the child with social taboos or behavioral issues which are not of immediate concern.

Adolescents and Young Adults

Unfortunately, sex education is often first introduced to students during puberty, when discussions of penises and vaginas cause an orchestra of giggling and a sea of red faces. The teacher's obvious embarrassment only makes everything worse.

Before individuals reach puberty, they should already know and understand the biological facts about reproduction and their own anatomy. However, a review of the facts is suggested to ensure that everyone has the right information. In one study, sexual education proved effective in delaying sexual intercourse among adolescents.

Needs. The primary thing adolescents need and crave is information about both the emotional and social aspects of sexual behavior. According to student polls, adolescents primarily desire information about (1) preparing for marriage and parenthood, (2) understanding and expressing their emotions, and (3) birth control. Pregnancy, sexually transmitted diseases, sexual performance, sexually related activities, homosexuality and alternative lifestyles, abortion, rape, sexual myths, sexual abuse, and values are other areas of concern and curiosity. Another thing pointed out by polls is that adolescents are very concerned with interaction skills and with issues of exploitation and assertiveness.

Unfortunately, most sex education programs stick to the cut-and-dried biological facts, and avoid the controversial issues which lie at the heart of sexuality and human behavior. Among certain populations, the issue of birth control needs to be addressed early, perhaps before the physical capability of conception develops. For example, in one study it was found that 20 percent of pregnant teenage girls became pregnant within the first month following loss of virginity.

Specific information regarding the whole spectrum of sexual activities must be provided, despite student claims that they know it all. Saying that AIDS is caused by sexual activity is not sufficient. Education such as this has led students to believe that AIDS is transmitted by kissing. All sexual activities need to be discussed.

Resistance Skills. Role playing is a useful technique among adolescents, whose identities and social abilities are always being challenged. In *role playing,* students act out situations in the classroom that mirror those the students often encounter in life.

In role playing, a student is faced with strong pressure to engage in wrongful sexual behavior, drug-related activities, or a number of other unhealthy or socially undesirable activities. In these play-acting situations, students practice their resistance skills, perhaps creating their own solutions or applying phrases or skills learned in the classroom. After each session, students and teacher discuss the session, evaluate both the effective and noneffective techniques, and relate the emotions aroused during the enactment.

Another technique particularly necessary for adolescents is called debriefing. *Debriefing* is particularly useful for countering the effects of movies, television, and the media. In debriefing, a person is reminded that the values, themes, or actions that are demonstrated in artificial media settings are not necessarily the values, themes, and actions of people in reality.

The resistance skills mentioned in the section on children are also useful for adolescents, with different twists. For example, an ally need not always be present, and adolescents can say "I promised my boyfriend/girlfriend I wouldn't."

Classroom Atmosphere. Sex education needs to take place in a supportive classroom environment. Educators must be nonjudgmental and encourage questions and comments from all participants. The qualities of empathy, openness, concern, respect, and trust are necessary.

Hopefully, the educator will help the students to share experiences, feelings, and opinions with one another, while recognizing different needs, allowing for different values, and guarding individual vulnerabilities.

Teachers should also open the door for private discussions with pupils.

Teachers. A teacher's ability to teach sex education does not seem to be related to age, sex, marital status, parental status, or religious or political orientation. Traits which apparently affect successful sex education are the teacher's beliefs about sex and the teacher's comfort with his or her own sexuality.

According to poll results, most teachers consider only biological facts important, and rarely give weight to or teach the more controversial issues of emotional and social aspects of sexual behavior, sexual performance, and birth control. Teachers tend to believe that the students' families are responsible for education of these issues.

Decision-Making Skills. Adolescence is a period when an individual's cognitive development is progressing from *concrete* to *abstract* operations. In childhood, an individual acquires the ability to perform concrete operations, mathematical functions, and to understand literal concepts — concepts that make sense to the eyes.

During adolescence, individuals generally develop the ability to perform abstract operations, which requires the understanding and application of theories—concepts which cannot be seen with the eyes. Answers are not specific words or numbers, but subjective responses. In regard to making decisions concerning their health, adolescents with better abstract thinking abilities are able to make better decisions concerning healthy behavior, particularly under stress.

Abstract thinking and decision making have three components: knowledge, skill, and action. Educational programs can introduce these components to adolescents and give them the opportunity to practice using them.

Prevention of Pregnancy. A three-component sex education program, which included: (1) classroom education, (2) adolescent counseling, and (3) availability of medical and birth control resources at a clinic for adolescents, proved effective in delaying the age of first intercourse by almost 1 year among inner-city youths. In addition, students began attending the clinic soon after beginning sexual activity. Some evidence suggested that adolescent girls educated in sexual matters were better able to resist their boyfriends' demands, resulting in a later age of initial sexual activity. These findings are important because among the adolescent population, pregnancy often occurs during the female's early sexual experiences. This research has clear application to AIDS education.

The Problem. Parents and communities rarely support sex education programs which extend beyond the biological facts. Strong negative community attitudes continue to blindfold children. Part of the problem stems from the desire of parents to control their children's sexual and social values, while relying on the educational system for other aspects of education and socialization. Unfortunately, adequate sexual and social knowledge is not always provided by the parents. In these instances, is society justified in stepping in and providing adequate education?

Homosexual Males

Homosexual males are a diverse group with varied educational needs. Because of the uniquely stressful situation many homosexual men now find themselves in, a few generalized comments can be made.

A significant proportion of homosexual men who engage in high-risk activities, such as multiple sex partners and anal intercourse, can benefit from educational and counseling efforts. Homosexual males need accurate, nonjudgmental information on HIV transmission, AIDS prevention, sexual hygiene, healthy living habits, and many aspects of AIDS itself. Socially, homosexual peer groups must encourage responsible sexual activity; such encouragement is already demonstrated in many communities. Psychologically, many homosexual males would benefit from counseling on life and death issues. Although many gay organizations and AIDS service organizations offer AIDS education, it is a mistake to assume that all homosexual males know the facts about AIDS.

A recent study performed by the Gay Men's Health Crisis in New York hints at the effectiveness of sexual education. Well-educated homosexual males in monogamous relationships improved their adherence to the rules of sexual hygiene after (1) having a medical overview, (2) participating in group risk-reduction programs, and (3) being shown explicit videos that encourage safe-sex activities.

IV Drug Users

IV drug users are a special group. These individuals often have major medical, social, and psychological needs.

Educational efforts aimed at IV drug users must first focus on stopping HIV transmission. The camaraderie of drug users should not be overlooked. Peer pressure might be effective. Counseling must work on building social skills for dealing with problems and stress while bringing drug use under control. Usually, IV drug users have specific nutritional and medical needs. They generally also need remedial education and job skill training.

Reportedly, the education of IV drug users is most successful when the students can identify with the teachers, that is, when teachers are ex-drug users or ex-convicts. Unfortunately, most public health departments refuse to hire people with such experience.

The Detroit Health Department, when attempting to communicate with the IV drug user population, found that their staff did not know or understand the beliefs and attitudes of the target population. As an alternative strategy, they encouraged members of high-risk groups to assume the leadership role, and to educate themselves and others. Relative success was also achieved with cooperative efforts between target populations and public health professionals.

Health Care Workers

Unfortunately, many health care workers still obtain the majority of their AIDS information from television, radio, newspapers, and general-interest magazines. While the media does fill in certain information gaps, it often does not present information in proper context, and does not dispel myths.

Health care workers need specific guidelines for and instruction in appropriate infection control procedures. The issue of noncompliance to rules and regulations needs to be tackled, with constant educational reinforcement, and probably peer pressure as well.

Homophobic and addict-phobic attitudes should be overcome through education. Health care workers need education about issues concerning alternative lifestyles, and need instruction on developing techniques to overcome the anxieties induced by these concepts. Some health care workers may require psychological counseling if fears develop into phobias.

15. AIDS in the Workplace

Employees with AIDS

The consensus is that a seropositive employee can perform normal duties as long as he or she is mentally and physically able. According to the current medical consensus on AIDS transmission, there is no need to restrict any seropositive person from using telephones, office equipment, toilets, showers, eating facilities, and water fountains.

If an infected person develops mental or physical problems which interfere with his or her ability to maintain infection control, then it is best to reevaluate the employee's status with all concerned parties, namely, management, union, medical counsel, public health personnel, and the employee.

Employee rights may be affected by federal, state, county, or city laws. Check with local state, county, or city health departments for applicable laws. Local AIDS service organizations may also have relevant information on hand. On the whole, court rulings have upheld the infected worker's right to work.

Conditions Which May Prevent Working

When an employee has a problem that interferes with infection control, the employee's medical status should be evaluated and a determination of the employment situation made. This process needs to be performed on a case-by-case basis, as jobs differ in their demands.

Conditions which may prevent an infected person from working are neurological symptoms preventing adequate mental function or lack of control of body functions: diarrhea, vomiting, lack of control over urine or bowel movements, uncoverable oozing wounds, nose bleeds, and biting or other violent behavior. Fatigue has been the major problem affecting the working capacity of HIV-infected people.

Employee Confidentiality

In the medical and public health communities the general trend is to protect the patient's privacy. Applicable federal, state, and local laws may apply. Employee and patient privacy laws, worker compensation regulations, employee civil rights, the confidentiality of medical records, and the issue of informed consent are also considerations in evaluating legal protection of confidentiality. Union and collective bargaining agreements may also play a role in these issues. The bottom line is that the employer and employee need to know the local statutes.

Confidentiality is an issue worth noting because its legal status may change.

For the Manager

The presence of a seropositive person in a working environment may affect internal discipline. The best way to avoid the fear of AIDS is to (1) educate the work force about AIDS transmission, and (2) institute a policy concerning seropositive employees and announce it even before such an individual appears.

It is best to let seropositive employees know that they are supported by policy and by applicable laws. Let them know how federal, state, county, and city laws and departmental rules will affect them. Explain that decisions concerning their employment will be made according to medical opinion, legal definitions, and management policies. Emphasize that control is not in the hands of fearful co-workers or the public. Discuss the issue of confidentiality. It is best to inquire about their work situation and their feelings about the situation and the job.

It may be necessary to move the seropositive person or change his or her tasks. Contact with many people or working on communal telephones puts an immunosuppressed person at risk of opportunistic infections.

Be watchful for harassment. It may be necessary to move the employee to an area where harassment can be controlled. Harassment can easily lead to legal problems. A harassed employee may desire a transfer. Be sensitive to transfer requests. Also consider altering work schedules and assignments.

According to current medical and public health consensus, AIDS is not transmitted in casual social contact. Thus any worker who refuses to work with a seropositive person may be subject to disciplinary measures and due process. However, a legal ruling found a prison worker to be improperly discharged because he refused to "pat down" an infected prisoner. The employee was considered improperly discharged because he had not received adequate education regarding HIV transmission.

The National Labor Relations Act (NLRA) possibly offers legal protection for employees refusing to work. The NLRA reportedly applies to most hospitals, profit and nonprofit. The NLRA protects employees who refuse to work because they have a reasonable belief that working conditions are not safe. Reasonable belief is open to interpretation.

Special Work Environments

Personal Service. Personal service workers are people who work in close physical contact with clients in a nonmedical or health care setting. Examples of personal service workers are barbers, hairdressers, cosmetologists, manicurists, pedicurists, massage therapists, and estheticians.

No known cases of nonsexual HIV transmission have occurred between a personal service worker and a client. Personal service workers who use sharp instruments should use the same precautions taken by health care workers. Blood spills are discussed in Chapter 19.

Personal service workers should be well educated in the transmission of HIV and all blood-borne infections. Education should stress the principles of good hygiene and disinfection. Seropositive personal service workers should not be restricted from working with clients; however, any personal service workers with bleeding or oozing dermatitis or skin wounds should not have contact with clients.

Food Service. Food service workers are people who are involved in the preparation or serving of food or beverages. Examples of food service workers are cooks, caterers, servers, waiters, bartenders, and airline attendants.

According to the CDC, all laboratory and epidemiological evidence suggests that blood-borne diseases and sexually transmitted diseases cannot be transmitted through preparation or serving of food or beverages. There are no known instances of either hepatitis B or HIV being transmitted through food.

Food service workers should exercise care to avoid injury to their hands. If a blood accident occurs, any food contaminated with blood should be discarded and the environment cleansed according to directions regarding blood spills in Chapter 19.

Seropositive food service workers should not be restricted from working; however, any food service workers with weeping dermatitis or skin wounds should not be allowed to handle food.

Acupuncture. No known cases of HIV infection have been transmitted by acupuncture needles. Acupuncture needles should be sterilized between uses. Acupuncturists should be well educated in the transmission of HIV and all blood-borne infections.

Tattooing. There have been media reports of a possible HIV transmission from tattooing. Tattooing needles are blood-letting instruments and should be sterilized between clients. Blood spills should be cleaned up appropriately. Tattooists should be well educated in the transmission of HIV and all blood-borne infections.

Ear Piercing. Ear-piercing needles are potentially blood-letting instruments. Even with no sign of blood, these needles should be sterilized or discarded after use. For disposal, place needles in a puncture-proof container such as a plastic pill bottle with a screw-on lid.

16. AIDS in Prisons

Experience has shown that guards and service personnel may be more concerned about AIDS than inmates. Because of their lifestyles, many inmates already know more about AIDS than the prison staff. Also, inmates may worry less about nonimmediate danger and uncertainty, and many may be more understanding of people in trouble.

Staff

Policy. Ideally, a written policy should be established and distributed prior to the appearance of a seropositive employee or inmate. Employees should be able to work as long as they are physically able and as long as they present no infection control problems.

Education. Prison staff need to be well educated regarding the facts of HIV transmission. They need to know when risk is present and when it is not. This education needs to be constantly reinforced. Even after initial AIDS education sessions, a California prison found it necessary to have AIDS-related 15-minute muster periods before each shift. In more formal settings question-and-answer periods were accompanied by special videotapes about AIDS made for law enforcement personnel.

Written information about AIDS and AIDS transmission should be made available in employee areas, such as the locker area and lunchroom. Training bulletins and department newsletters may also devote space to AIDS education.

Confidentiality. Confidentiality is a difficult issue in prisons. Guards want to know who is infected, and this may be justified in some instances. Inmates are often the first to discover who is seropositive or ill.

Risk. Guards are at risk. Some degree of risk is unavoidable, considering the working environment and their tasks. At any time, guards may be exposed to a number of contaminated substances. A fight or struggle may expose them to blood, saliva, or nasal secretions. Inmates have been known to throw feces at guards. Guards must also search cells, and they sometimes discover hidden IV needles by being stuck with them. Inmates also use safety pins to puncture veins and eye droppers to inject drugs.

Inmate Isolation. Generally, isolation of seropositive inmates seems unnecessary, although it is practiced. Inmates who maintain infection control standards present little risk to guards and other inmates. Inmate hospitalization has been practiced for the sake of convenience rather than out of medical necessity. Separate housing for large numbers of seropositive inmates has been considered for inmate control reasons, rather than for infection control reasons. Some debate exists whether or not this is feasible. At least two legal rulings support prison officials in their decision to segregate inmates with AIDS.

Inmates

Testing Inmates. Officials must decide whether or not to routinely screen prisoners for HIV infection and how to best inform inmates and the necessary personnel. Federal, state, city, and county statutes may affect screening and confidentiality.

The federal prison system has performed a test of prisoners and has found low levels of the virus. The federal prison system is not representative of the prison systems of all states; the types of prisoners and the crimes they commit vary. IV drug users are more likely to be found in local prison systems, depending on the geographic locale. A minority of states have instituted mandated screening programs. Most states selectively screen prisoners. Some prisoners request AIDS testing to confirm a diagnosis or after a rape.

Testing does not solve the problem of what to do with an infected prisoner. The confidentiality statutes vary from state to state. Reportedly, some infected prisoners have been released without notification of local health authorities and without any counseling or medical support.

Inmate Education. Inmates need to be well educated with the facts about HIV transmission and provided with the proper equipment for prevention. A variety of approaches was attempted in California, but the most successful were group classes on AIDS run by the prison's medical personnel. The classes using videotapes and films were the most popular. Pamphlets and posters on AIDS and AIDS transmission were also made available to inmates. Inmate newspapers featured articles on AIDS education.

IV Drug Use. IV drug use is a serious problem in prisons. Some kind of compromise should be reached which recognizes the fact that contraband hypodermic needles or their substitutes do exist.

Tattooing. Prisoners use pins, pens, and other sharp instruments to create homemade tattoos. Prisoners should be warned that if they share these instruments with other inmates, a risk of HIV transmission exists.

Razors. Razors are potential weapons. Formerly, several prisoners would shave with one razor blade locked into its holder. This practice should be discontinued in favor of disposable razors.

Condoms. While some prison systems distribute condoms to inmates, many systems will not. Prevention of AIDS in the prison population must include the use of condoms.

17. AIDS in Schools

The issue of AIDS in schools is emotionally charged. Many ongoing legal battles exist over the school attendance of seropositive children. The same is true regarding the employment of homosexual teachers and HIV-infected teachers. Although a legal consensus will eventually evolve, a process of precedent-setting is currently under way. The legal history of AIDS is still too short to make broad statements regarding student or teacher rights. In the short term, court decisions may vary by state, region, or community.

Seropositive students have been barred, at least temporarily, from schools. When these policies are challenged in court, the courts usually decide in favor of allowing the HIV-infected child to attend school. One judge even ordered the readmittance of a seropositive student who bit another student, citing the 1973 handicap law, which orders school districts to accommodate students' handicaps. These rulings are similar to those in cases of students infected with herpes and hepatitis B who have been allowed to attend school.

Suggested Recommendations

The following recommendations have been established by the National Education Association (NEA) and the Centers for Disease Control (CDC). Such recommendations do not have the power of law.

Both staff and students need to be educated in the facts regarding HIV transmission. Policies regarding HIV-infected students and employees should be created and distributed before any HIV-infected person appears. A special staffperson or counselor knowledgeable about sexual matters, including homosexuality, AIDS, and how to deal with seropositive patients should be available. Alternatively, an association with local AIDS service groups may be formed.

The NEA concludes in its recommendations that school officials may request that a student or employee submit to HIV testing, provided that the school officials have reasonable cause to suspect the person is at high risk for HIV infection. The NEA states that the sexual orientation of the student or employee shall not constitute reasonable cause for a person to be suspected of HIV infection. According to NEA recommendations, no student, employee, or potential employee need provide information on his or her sexual orientation. Testing of all students and employees is not perceived as necessary by most public health officials.

The CDC and NEA both agree that seropositive students, as long as they are physically and mentally able to function in the classroom and maintain infection control, should not be placed in restricted settings. Seropositive students need not be restricted from classroom activities, public bathrooms, or cafeterias.

The CDC suggests the same guidelines for preschool-age children, again as long as open lesions are not present and as long as the child has appropriate self-control. However, it might not be wise for seropositive children to attend day care centers. Outbreaks of cytomegalovirus (CMV), a suspected co-factor of AIDS, are known to occur in day care centers. CMV is easily transmitted. (See Figure 10.)

Conditions which could remove a student from a nonrestricted setting might include: neurological handicaps or problems; lack of body control; lack of control over bowel movements or urine retention; displays of biting or other violent behavior; and the presence of uncoverable, oozing lesions. Careful monitoring of an HIV-infected child is very important for many reasons, including the facts that the neurological symptoms can be severe and progress rapidly, certain milestones in behavioral and cognitive development may never be reached.

Seropositive employees should not be restricted from work or school activities except when conditions mentioned above or an infection control problem disallow it.

In the event of these or other problems, the student's or employee's status should be determined on a case-by-case basis by a team consisting of public health personnel, physicians, the students' parents, and the appropriate school personnel. Considerations evaluated by the team might include the behavioral, neurological, and physical condition of the student or employee, the type of interaction the infected person has with teachers and students, and the impact of the infected person's presence on others.

If the student is not able to attend regular classes, the NEA recommends that every reasonable effort be made to provide adequate alternative education; any school personnel involved in such efforts should be volunteers.

If an employee is not able to work, the NEA recommends that every available effort be made to place the employee on medical leave and begin disability benefits.

The NEA also recommends that the identity of the student or employee not be publicly revealed. Only personnel who have close personal contact with an infected student or employee need have knowledge of the seropositivity.

For more information on recommendations regarding the education of HIV-infected children, see Appendix B. The information may also be of interest to professionals concerned with infection control.

Risky Behaviors

Tattooing, ear piercing, and becoming blood brothers are common childhood and adolescent group activities. The use of illegal steroids by body builders and athletes and the sharing of those needles is common. IV drug use is also found in some high school populations. These activities need to be discouraged, with proper explanations as to the AIDS risks involved. In addition, methods of infection control, such as bleach sterilization, may be taught.

Lice Control

Head lice are sometimes a problem among school-age children and adolescents. Although the risk of insect transmission of HIV is probably very low, lice are suspected of transmitting a variety of bacterial infections and are a vehicle for the transmission of typhus from rats to humans.

Periodically, students at schools should be screened for lice; all students should be screened. Lice often travel from one person to another in hats, combs, and perhaps scarves; therefore, students should be informed that these items are personal and are not to be shared.

More information on lice and lice control is available from the National Pediculosis Association, P.O Box 149, Newton, MA 02161. (617) 449-NITS.

18. AIDS and the Law

AIDS presents an extremely difficult challenge to law and justice because as far as AIDS is concerned, law and science are advancing at different rates. The study of AIDS encompasses many different scientific disciplines, all evolving at their own pace. In the same manner, the legal issues surrounding AIDS are diverse, and disputes exist in many aspects of public and private life.

Once a law is written, the courts have to decide how to interpret it justly. In practice, legal decisions in the court are strongly influenced by precedents. Precedents are previous court decisions made on cases of a nature similar to the case under immediate consideration. Courts are currently creating many AIDS-related legal precedents.

Court decisions may vary from region to region and community to community. Local city, county, or state public health departments and local AIDS service organizations may have region-specific legal information.

The information presented here is not to be construed as legal counsel.

Discrimination

Employment. The earliest legal disputes over AIDS concerned HIV-infected people in occupational settings.

AIDS was defined as a handicap under the Vocational Rehabilitation Act of 1973 by a federal judge hearing a case. A handicap is defined as a mental or physical impairment which substantially limits one or more of a person's major life activities. Whether this ruling will hold true for all AIDS cases in the future remains to be seen.

At least forty-two states and Washington, D.C. have laws that prohibit discrimination against the handicapped. The Vocational Rehabilitation Act of 1973 prohibits discrimination toward federal employees and in any federally funded program, grant, or project. Various local jurisdictions are amending or enacting local ordinances to prevent or reduce AIDS-related discrimination.

Generally, courts have upheld the right of the HIV-infected worker to work. Several decisions have awarded money reimbursement to individuals wrongly discharged from work. A major legal battle, yet to be decisively determined, is the barring of seropositive teachers from schools. School board policies are being challenged by virtually every special interest group concerned about AIDS.

Few regions have regulations which prevent discrimination on the basis of homosexuality. In most regions of the United States, an employer is able to discharge an employee because the employee is a homosexual.

Also, in some regions, an employer has the right to demand medical examinations as a condition of employment—a concern to HIV-infected individuals. Generally, this request can be made only after employment has been offered.

Housing. Many seropositive and ill people have been evicted from their apartments by landlords or roommates. If the handicap and disability definition of AIDS holds, then it may offer legal protection under housing discrimination laws found in many states. A few legislators in California have tried to make it mandatory for realtors to inform potential buyers when the previous owner of a house or apartment died of AIDS. At least one realty group has made this an internal policy.

Hospitals. Hospitals have refused to treat AIDS patients. This practice will probably become less frequent in the future. Initially, smaller rural hospitals referred all AIDS patients to larger more experienced urban hospitals. Sometimes this referral kept critically ill AIDS patients in emergency rooms for hours or days before they were transferred scores of miles away via ambulance.

Generally, hospitals are not required to treat patients without the mutual consent of both the hospital and the patient. However, hospitals receiving federal funds cannot refuse to treat patients on a discriminatory basis. Hospitals cannot refuse to treat a patient in an emergency, but this emergency status is open to interpretation. A patient may be transferred to an appropriate facility as long as the transfer does not delay treatment.

Once a hospital has accepted a patient, it is legally required to care for the patient. The hospital has the legal duty to provide its employees with the necessary equipment and the appropriate policies and procedures to safely care for the patient—safe for the patient, safe for the employees, and safe for the hospital's other patients.

The Centers for Disease Control publishes a series of recommendations for health care and allied professionals. Hospitals are not required to adopt CDC guidelines into their own procedures and policies; however, they may obtain some legal protection by doing so. If a hospital adopts CDC guidelines, it could be difficult to prove that the hospital failed to meet the standard of care for preventing HIV transmission, provided these guidelines are followed.

Nurses and other health care professionals have refused to care for AIDS patients. There is some dispute over the legal rights of an employee to make such a refusal and of employers to discharge such employees. If a nurse or other hospital employee refused to treat an AIDS patient and patient injury resulted, then the nurse might be found negligent and liable. A court or jury decision in such a case would be based on whether or not the employee's refusal was reasonable.

Other Services. In most states, stores, restaurants, funeral homes, and other public accommodations and businesses are not allowed to discriminate, because of disability laws. Individuals who provide services might be allowed to discriminate.

Reporting

Reporting requirements for AIDS cases and other infectious diseases are established separately by each state. Nearly all states require the reporting of communicable disease cases, such as AIDS. Generally, physicians, laboratories, hospitals, and other persons who know about or attend to a communicable disease case must report the case to the county or state health department. Fines for failure to do so range from $5 to $1000; jail sentences can extend up to 90 days.

In Fall 1987, the following states had mandatory reporting of any seropositive test result: Arizona, Colorado, Georgia, Minnesota, Nevada, and South Carolina. Most states require reporting of CDC-defined AIDS cases. A few states still have voluntary reporting of AIDS.

Confidentiality

Most federal and state health agencies recommend that the identities of seropositive people remain confidential or be known to only a select group. To date, only California has created a law which specifically protects the confidentiality of HIV test results. In California, disclosure of a person's AIDS test results is illegal without the written authorization of the patient.

Because of human nature, there are never any absolute guarantees of confidentiality in anything. However, in one legal challenge, confidentiality was maintained. In Florida, a transfusion recipient of fifty-one units of blood was not able to obtain the names of blood donors at the local blood bank. The names were requested in order to link the recipient's HIV infection to the blood transfusions; confidentiality won out over the plaintiff's right to the information.

Finally, several lawsuits for defamation have come about because individuals have communicated falsely by written or oral means that a patient had AIDS. Defamation is the wrongful injury of a person's reputation.

AIDS Research. Many HIV-infected people are taking part in AIDS-related scientific studies. At the federal level the Protection of Human Subject Regulations protect the confidentiality of human subjects participating in the majority of research conducted by the U.S. Department of Health and Human Services. Participants in such federally funded studies sign informed-consent forms, which describe the intended use, distribution, and confidentiality of the information gathered for the study. Most AIDS research conducted by the CDC is protected by the Public Health Service Act, which stringently protects any epidemiological information collected by the Centers for Disease Control.

Contact Tracing. With STDs in the past, doctors or health departments were considered responsible for tracking down the sexual partners of STD-infected people and for ensuring that the partners received medical treatment. After the development of penicillin and other miracle drugs, less and less effort went into contact tracing. Miracle drugs made STDs easy to treat, and it was thought that uncontacted sexual partners would eventually seek treatment on their own.

With AIDS, contact tracing is still an evolving issue. Voluntary tracing is strongly encouraged by the U.S. Public Health Service. However, certain offices and individuals in federal and state health departments are seeking mandatory contact tracing. Currently, the report of an AIDS case to a public health department does not mean that contact tracing occurs. In some areas, only heterosexual contacts are tracked down, since heterosexuals consider themselves at a lower risk than homosexuals. It is the opinion of some public health officials that homosexuals, particularly in urban areas, realize the extent of their risk, are more knowledgeable about AIDS, and are more likely to be aware that they are at risk, or that a past sexual partner is at risk.

Liability

Individual. There appears to be a growing consensus that individuals are responsible for informing their sex partners about their health status concerning STDs. In one liability suit an individual's homeowner insurance company had to pay damages to a woman because the male homeowner had allegedly given her herpes.

There are a growing number of criminal assault charges involving seropositive people. One soldier is currently being court-martialed for the equivalent of assault for allegedly having sex with two women and one man without informing them of his seropositive status. In another case, a seropositive prisoner has been charged with criminal assault because he allegedly tried to bite law enforcement officers.

Physicians. Concerning their patients, physicians are obligated to keep all nonreportable facts confidential. Any breach of this confidence on the part of the physician may expose him or her to the risk of lawsuits for wrongful disclosure. Claims may be made by patients for damages. In California, at least one lawsuit is pending on the disclosure of a person's AIDS test results without the written authorization of the patient.

Physicians are also required to explain fully to seropositive patients the currently accepted view as to the best methods of infection control. Some question exists whether or not it is unlawful for a physician or a public health department official to breach patient confidentiality in order to warn the patient's sex partners or spouse that the patient is seropositive. The consensus, though not conclusive, seems to lean toward informing those known without question to be at risk.

If an AIDS case or an infectious disease case results from a physician's failure to report the case to public health authorities, then the physician may be liable for damages. In addition, the physican's license may be in jeopardy. These lawsuits are an extension of the individual liability themes previously mentioned. An injured party, the one who catches AIDS or any STD, may sue a solvent third party, if the third party had previous knowledge that the culprit was infected. A growth in the number of cases directed against knowledgeable third parties is expected.

Blood Transfusions. A number of lawsuits have been filed primarily against blood banks and blood product manufacturers because of transfusion-related AIDS.

In nearly all states, supplying blood is considered to be a service rather than a product. Thus, court decisions have not held to the standards of traditional strict product liability. In short, plaintiffs have not been able to collect. These decisions may or may not hold.

Blood transfusions, as a service, are generally held to be as safe as technologically possible. At the time most blood-related cases of HIV transmission took place, there was no available technique for detecting the presence of HIV in blood.

In order for a person to collect money for damages in a lawsuit concerning blood-borne HIV transmission, he or she must show that the blood supplier was negligent. In one such case, a blood bank settled out of court because an administrative error allowed blood from an infected donor to be used in a hospital transfusion.

State Police Powers

As part of their police powers, states are able to quarantine individuals or otherwise exercise their authority in order to control the spread of communicable diseases. Historically, these police powers have been exercised with diseases such as smallpox, yellow fever, and cholera—diseases which can only be transmitted at certain stages of infection, usually an acute period lasting a number of days or weeks.

HIV infection presents a different problem. First, it is transmitted primarily by sexual contact, IV drug use, or by blood; behaviors which generally require the consent of participants. Second, no one knows at what stage or stages of infection HIV is transmissible.

Inevitably, some HIV-infected patients are irresponsible in their behavior. It is generally considered necessary and desirable to institute compulsory quarantine procedures where voluntary measures do not work. However, the least restrictive measures should be attempted first.

In a few instances HIV-infected people have been quarantined. One such case involved a prostitute in Florida who was ordered to carry a radio monitor, which signaled when she strayed too far from her home. Another case involved a homosexual male who continued to work as a prostitute despite his seropositivity. This case revealed the problems of restraint since quarantine authority did not directly reside with the police, who detained him. This particular situation was resolved when the local homosexual community provided the man with a place to stay and promised responsible supervision.

In a different application of police powers, the cities of New York and San Francisco placed restrictions on homosexual bathhouses operating in their cities and closed those bathhouses and other places which promoted anonymous homosexual activity.

In Nevada, all prostitutes in county-licensed brothels must be tested for HIV and other STDs as a condition of employment. In Florida, convicted prostitutes are tested for STDs and HIV.

Immigration

The Department of Health and Human Services has the authority to act to prevent the spread of disease across state and national borders. Generally, it relies on individual states to act under their own powers. AIDS will soon be added to the list of diseases for which a person can be quarantined.

People who are not U.S. citizens can be prevented from entering the United States if they have dangerous contagious diseases. AIDS will soon be added to the list of diseases. Foreigners entering the United States must submit to medical examination upon request.

Insurance Testing

The AIDS epidemic developed very quickly for the insurance industry. Suddenly, insurance companies had to pay a number of expensive medical claims for this new disease. Since AIDS is not calculated into the current pricing structure of insurance, the insurance companies found themselves losing money on a factor not previously considered. Whether the insurance industry can afford to do this or not is a matter of some debate.

Nevertheless, insurance companies wish to test certain people who are applying for health, medical, or life insurance. Also some insurance companies wish to write restrictions into their policies, so that a person cannot receive payments for AIDS-related problems for the first 2 years of the policy.

Insurance companies are heavily regulated by state governments. Thus far, a handful of states have passed laws preventing testing by insurance companies, limiting the use or release of this information by insurance companies, or limiting the disclosure of testing results by physicians. The future holds many legal and political battles over this issue.

Mortuaries

CDC recommends that HIV-infected bodies be identified for the benefit of undertakers. CDC recommendations are not legally binding. Some lawsuits have arisen because funeral homes have refused to embalm HIV-infected bodies.

Emergency Medical Technicians (EMTs)

Some states have altered confidentiality laws to require that medical facilities notify EMTs within 48 hours of diagnosis that a patient they transferred has an infectious disease.

19. The Challenge for Medical Professionals

Medical professionals are trained to handle deadly and infectious diseases and treat patients afflicted with such diseases. Yet medical professionals are human and subject to human fears. Fear grows rapidly in the absence of accurate information, or specific instructions, protocols, and policies. Given the proper information and guidelines, most health care professionals can gain the confidence to provide quality care to the AIDS patient.

Health Care Workers

The information provided here is gathered from many sources. While this information is not to be construed as a guideline or recommendation, it is intended to help those responsible for care and infection control as well as make others aware of the issues. Appendix C lists CDC recommendations for prevention of HIV transmission in the workplace.

The Nightmare. In many ways, health care workers are a special group. Many individual health care workers made sacrifices to obtain their credentials and they place great pride in their education and profession. Yet the care some AIDS patients have received, and perhaps are still receiving, has the aspect of a nightmare, or a setting out of the Middle Ages.

The medical horrors listed here occurred primarily in large urban hospitals during the beginning of the AIDS epidemic, but these behaviors are continuing to spread into smaller rural hospitals as the distribution of AIDS cases increases. These examples demonstrate the need for proper protocols, policies, and procedures in medical settings.

Severely ill AIDS patients have been left waiting in emergency rooms for 8 to 12 hours, in one case for 3 days, until a single-bed hospital room became available. The consensus opinion in the medical community is that AIDS patients do not need private rooms, barring uncontrollable behavior or diarrhea.

Severely ill patients have been refused treatment at hospitals and, in non-stable conditions, transported to hospitals scores of miles distant. Ambulances have refused to transport AIDS patients, technicians have refused to draw their blood, anesthesiologists (who put people to sleep for operations), surgeons, and pathologists (who examine dead bodies) have refused to perform their specialized tasks. Psychiatrists and counselors have refused to counsel AIDS patients.

Once admitted to the hospital, some AIDS patients were not allowed to see their lovers, family, or friends, given little or inaccurate information concerning their health status, denied use of bathrooms and telephones, and had their confidentiality breached, as gossip of their health status rushed through the hospital like wildfire.

Most health care workers cringe at the thought of the following tragedies.

Yet they all have occurred and may still be occurring: patient calls left unanswered; food trays left at the doors of rooms of patients who were unable to move; oxygen humidifiers allowed to run dry; patients left unbathed who were bedridden and unable to control urine or bowel movements while ulcers and blisters formed on their skin; blood-encrusted intravenous tubing left in swollen and infected arms; parents and friends forced to search the hospital for clean linen and clothes for the patient; the patients' clothes and personal possessions burned. Also, patients have been denied information about test results, discharged, and denied medical advice and information on how to prevent HIV transmission.

Fear. Most health care professionals have AIDS-related fears of contagion and death. Such fear is natural: AIDS is a fearful thing. It is a disease which kills, but often not before causing blindness, deafness, paralysis, dementia, and horrifying weight loss. While caring for HIV-infected patients, even minor, common occupational accidents, such as sticking oneself with a used hypodermic needle, become life-and-death concerns for the health care professional. While fear is natural and can be harnessed to promote appropriate infection control procedures, individuals and management must strive to prevent fear from developing into phobia.

AIDS-related anxiety usually arises from the staff's self-perceived lack of knowledge concerning AIDS. Anxiety is increased by the unknown nature of AIDS and insecurity regarding infection control procedures. For the most part, health care workers do have adequate knowledge of appropriate infection control procedures—hepatitis B procedures are more than adequate—and merely need this knowledge reinforced.

Fear, which can lead to patient abuse, can be countered with facts. Education is the best way to deal with fear, because accurate facts remove irrational concerns and promote appropriate behavior where risks are present. Health care workers need to be well versed in the matters of AIDS transmission and infection control procedures.

Phobia. A phobia is an irrational fear or dislike of something. In a phobia, fear is so extreme that it interferes with the functioning of the individual. Phobias are thought to occur when individuals, subconsciously, focus all their fears on one object. This phenomenon is sometimes called *countertransference* or *displacement* in psychology.

A strong tendency to stereotype patients exists in too many staffs. It is possible that some of the fear exhibited by health care workers is not based on fear of contagion. Rather, these health care workers might fear homosexuals and drug users whether the patient is one or not. These fears have been called "homophobia" and "addict-phobia." These phobias can lead to apathy on the part of the caregiver, a possible cause of patient neglect and abuse.

Several recent studies have centered on health care worker attitudes toward homosexuality. The most striking result of one study was that health care workers' attitudes toward AIDS patients were not related to health care workers' knowledge of AIDS. Rather, worker attitudes toward AIDS patients were linked to attitudes about homosexuality. In other words, a professional's fear of an AIDS patient may not be caused by fear of AIDS, but by fear of the lifestyle represented by the patient.

Some psychologists suggest that homosexuals and drug users are the targets of phobias because medical professionals do not fear disease as much as they fear that the stigma of these unpopular groups might rub off on them. Health care workers receive more community appreciation and respect from caring for the mayor than for the local drunk. In addition, some mental health professionals suggest that medical staff members fear the illicit impulses that nontraditional individuals represent; that is, the health care worker fears that some of these people's "evil" will rub off on them.

This information indicates that, in certain regions, AIDS educational programs for health care workers must combat such phobias and be designed to create empathy for alternative lifestyles. If a phobia adversely affects a person's occupational functioning, then counseling might be suggested in an attempt to bring to light the issues behind the phobia.

Phobias need not be focused on the patient. In other displacement problems, health care workers or other individuals develop phobias concerning fear of contagion which focus on bathrooms or public objects, such as magazines or doorknobs.

Burnout. Reports of health care worker burnout are common. Burnout occurs when people are so drained by their work that their efficiency suffers. Worker health may suffer too. Nurses, who spend more time with patients than any other medical professionals, are particularly susceptible to burnout.

Caring for AIDS patients is emotionally difficult. First, the effects of the disease are awful to watch. Second, most AIDS patients are in the prime of their lives, often age-peers of the health care providers. Many health care workers are accustomed to seeing old people die. But seeing the death of large numbers of young people can produce deep and powerful emotions within the health care provider. In addition, the actual care of the AIDS patient is stressful even in a purely professional sen: AIDS presents difficult legal, administrative, and ethical problems, all boosting the stress level of the medical professional.

Moreover, a larger number of medical professionals—born, raised, and educated in an era when infectious disease seemed defeated—must now face new limitations. They are greatly distressed by not being able to cure the patient, and must accept a new role as merely a reliever of pain.

All these issues affect morale, and morale affects the quality of care. As much as possible, steps should be taken to avoid burnout or lessen its impact. To avoid burnout as much as possible, the individual health care worker should pay close attention to his or her own physical and emotional health, making sure that he or she continues to balance life's needs and activities.

Emotional outlets must be created for the mental and emotional health of highly stressed health care workers. A time and place should be set aside so they can openly discuss their fears, concerns, and emotions, as well as exchange notes about better care and clear the air over grievances and protocols. Professional counseling might be made available, or health care workers might form support groups, or some other arrangements might be made. Some experimentation in this area will be necessary to find out what methods work.

Overcompensation. Health care worker reactions to the extraordinary stress associated with AIDS vary. Overcompensation, called *reaction formation* in psychology, is a frequent response seen in dedicated staff members. Reaction formation is expressed in many different ways and seems to stem from the health care worker's difficulty in establishing a safe emotional distance from patients. At one end of the spectrum, the health care worker identifies too strongly with the patient, and thus suffers the slow death of a friend. In a similar vein, the staff member may become the perfect caregiver, when in actuality he or she wants to run for the hills. Stress builds as the individual acts in opposition to his or her personal feelings. At the opposite end of the emotional spectrum, the health care worker withdraws to an emotional distance, appearing completely disinterested in the patient.

The Future. People become medical professionals for a number of reasons, ranging from a desire for financial security to a desire to perform a valuable community service. For young people considering health care as a profession, AIDS has changed their vision, regardless of their viewpoint.

AIDS has changed the educational experience of the young core of medical and nursing students now working in hospitals. In certain urban medical centers, AIDS dominates the time allotted to students for reading, conferences, and hospital rounds. In addition, the course of therapy for AIDS patients is controlled by research personnel, robbing the students of valuable experience in learning to make decisions. Students also lose experience in treating a wide variety of diseases and conditions, because their labor is necessarily devoted to AIDS management. This lack of experience may become evident in the future.

Patient Care

Patient Care Team. Because HIV and related infections and conditions cover such a broad spectrum of medical knowledge, many hospitals have adopted a team approach, mixing many different disciplines of medicine. Such a team might primarily include: (1) one or more physicians (often an internist and specialists in infectious disease, oncology, immunology, and dermatology); (2) nurses or nursing staff representative; (3) a social worker or staff representative; and perhaps, (4) a patient advocate. The medical professionals of this team evaluate the patient's medical, nursing, and social needs of both the patient and the patient's family. The patient advocate legally represents the wishes of the patient, who may not be mentally competent at all times during the course of the disease.

Additional consulting staff might include a psychiatrist, a psychiatric nurse, an infection control practitioner, alcohol or drug abuse counselors, and counselors who specialize in compulsive behaviors.

Naturally, team interaction needs to be continuous; one person may be the coordinator. Team discussions should cover medical issues as well as issues concerning alternative lifestyles, drug abuse, homosexuality, staff fears, staff grief, and burnout.

Ideally, team guidelines, roles, responsibilities, protocols, and procedures should be established before the need for the team arises.

Nursing Interventions. Now that more is known about AIDS, nurses are more able to attend to the needs of AIDS patients and to lessen their physical and mental suffering. Care must necessarily be individualized. Communication between the patient and the caregiver is of key importance. (See Figure 25.)

Patient-Based Infection Control. Health care workers must pay particular attention to factors in the care setting which expose seropositive patients to infection.

Pins and needles used to examine the patient for sensory perception should be used once and discarded in an appropriate container. HIV-infected patients might be assigned their own personal hygiene equipment, such as bowls, wash basins, and thermometers. It is suggested that single-use nebulizers (an apparatus which creates a fine mist) be used, and that patient masks, nasal suction tubes, and other tubing be replaced daily.

Invasive Procedures. Invasive procedures are defined as the surgical entry into tissues, cavities, or organs. These procedures might be performed in an operating room, delivery room, emergency department, or outpatient settings in both doctors' and dentists' offices.

To prevent HIV transmission during invasive procedures, it is suggested that all relevant health care workers be well educated in regard to HIV epidemiology, transmission, and proper infection control procedures, including the need for such appropriate barrier precautions as protective clothing. Health care workers with certain illnesses or conditions should not perform invasive procedures. Routine HIV screening of health care workers who perform invasive procedures is not generally recommended.

All health care workers should wear gloves when touching nonintact skin or mucous membranes, and use other protection, such as gowns, masks, goggles, or face shields, as necessary. Barrier precautions should be observed during invasive procedures and afterward until all instruments, equipment, and surfaces have been properly decontaminated or disposed of.

Extraordinary care must be used during cleaning, disposal, and handling of contaminated instruments. All sharp instruments should be placed in appropriate puncture-resistant containers. Plastic bottles with screw-on caps are suggested.

Due to the risk of infection, invasive procedures should be kept to a minimum in HIV-infected patients and used only when necessary. Suctioning should be performed with sterile catheters, gloves, and solutions. Urinary catheters should be used only when necessary; the same is true for intravenous therapy.

Isolation. Infection control procedures should isolate germs, not the patient. It is easy for an AIDS patient to become physically and emotionally isolated when treated purely as the origin of disease.

According to current thought, HIV-infected patients need not be isolated from other patients unless they have uncontrollable diarrhea or other conditions which might easily transmit infection. However, respiratory precautions must be observed in some instances. Immunosuppressed AIDS patients should not be placed in situations where they might catch an opportunistic infection

Figure 25: Nursing Interventions

Assessment.	Suggested assessments of AIDS patients include medical examination, evaluation of their nutritional status, exercise and rest regimens, levels and types of stress normally encountered, and an accounting of their stress management techniques, including alcohol, drugs and smoking. An assessment should be made of the patient's risk of encountering further doses of HIV and other STD's. Medical examination should overview the patient's status regarding presence of opportunistic infections, neurological function, cognitive function, pulmonary function, gastrointestinal function, urinary function, level of physical competency, status of the patient's skin, and pain. Standard psychiatric interviews and neuropsychiatric examinations are suggested for testing cognitive functions. Cognitive and psychological assessment should be ongoing. Careful social, sexual, and drug histories should be elicited with sensitive patient questioning and an acute ear. Punitive questioning should be avoided. Listening to the client's explanations may prevent stereotyping.
Autonomy.	There are two issues of autonomy. First, the patient should be given care in a non-coercive setting, fully aware of clinical procedures, potential dangers, test results, where and how the information regarding their health status will be distributed, and plans for medical care. Health care and information should be provided in a non-punitive fashion and provided in terms and language the person can understand. The patient should be able to make informed decisions concerning their own health care. HIV-infected people should also be encouraged to become involved in their own health care. The caregiver can aid the patient by helping him or her set reasonable limits on physical activities. Allowing the patient autonomy may require a conscious effort on the part of the caregiver. Health care workers *expect* the patient to be sick and to play the role of patient, so the health care worker can play the role of caregiver. The health care worker can subliminally enforce these roles, promoting patient stress. Whenever possible, in order to enhance the patient's autonomy, outpatient care and community involvement are suggested. Community resources may stem from family, friends, religious organizations, or AIDS-service organizations, which generally service all AIDS patients, not only homosexual males.
Bleach.	Bleach is a very strong chemical agent (oxidizer). Flush drains before and after use. Keep area well ventilated. *DO NOT mix bleach with other household or commercial cleaners* such as toilet bowl cleaners, rust removers, acid or ammonia containing products. If bleach is mixed with these substances, deadly gases may be chemically released.
Blood/Body-Fluid Precautions.	In a patient having blood/body-fluid precautions, all body fluids must be treated as potentially contaminated since all body fluids communicate with the blood. Health care workers should wear appropriate protective equipment when risk of exposure exists.

Diarrhea.	Diarrhea is life-threatening. Diarrhea can lead to dehydration and electrolyte imbalance, the latter potentially causing hallucinations. Encourage the patient to drink fluids, monitor patient bowel activity and fluid excretion; watch for signs of dehydration. Intravenous fluid therapy may be necessary.
Disorientation.	Provide visual clues for the disorientated patient, such as large clocks and calanders. Mark the bathroom, other rooms, and closets with signs. Talk frequently about family, friends, work, and common activities. Patients with serious neurological problems, such as advanced dementia, may require round-the-clock supervision.
Family Care.	Families of AIDS patients need care too. A health care worker may direct the families to local support groups, religious organizations, professional counseling, or other mental health resources.

The problems a family faces are: social isolation stemming from the social stigma of AIDS; a great financial burden; and, perhaps, the public disclosure of behaviors previously secret or denied. A common theme of homosexual males is a geographically-or emotionally-distant biological family replaced by a nearby extended family. The former may not tolerate the latter. Unless other measures have been taken, the biologic family may ban the extended family from the hospital, thus denying the patient his or her strongest emotional contacts.

A frequent finding is that the mother of homosexual males frequently blame themselves for the son's disease and his homosexuality, losing their faith in their parenting ability and threatening their self-image and sense of control. Counseling may be suggested. |
| **Hygiene.** | It is suggested that AIDS patients shower or bath daily to reduce the number of surface bacteria present. A mild soap and non-abrasive flannel cloth should used to work up a lather covering the body, followed by thorough rinsing and the application of body lotions, cream, or a thin layer of petroleum jelly to retain natural skin moisture. The skin should be examined carefully for skin lesions. This is a good time to examine the lymph nodes also.

For oral hygiene, every effort should be made to keep the mucous membranes and internal mouth surfaces intact. It is suggested that toothbrushing be avoided because it causes bleeding. Dental flossing and a thorough rinsing are suggested instead, although flossing can initially cause bleeding. Blood is a contaminated substance. It is suggested that an unconcious patient have his or her mouth cleaned three times daily with a gloved finger, gauze and a spatula.

With hairwashing, soaps containing alcohols should be avoided. Hair loss is a problem with anti-cancer chemotherapy so hairwashing in these patients might be limited to twice weekly or so, and silk caps or other nightcaps might be worn to prevent hair loss from friction of the head on the pillow.

Following voiding the rectal area should be cleaned to avoid potential infections from organisms living in feces. |

Incontinence.	Adult diapers are suggested for the incontinent patient, allowing the patient some independence. Condom catheters are suggested as preferable to indwelling catheters, the latter having a higher risk of introducing infection.
Nutrition.	Weight loss and malnutrition alter immune system function and may further reduce the patient's resistance to infections. While little is known about the mechanism or malnutrition in AIDS, some clinical counters to it can be attempted. It is suggested that food be presented to the patient frequently in small, visually appealing portions. The food should be high in nutritional status, high in caloric and protein value and low in residue. Nutrient-rich snacks like raisins and peanuts might be made available. Bland foods and foods at room temperature may be more comfortable for patients with oral lesions. Diarrhea may be controlled with anti-diarrheal agents and a diet low in residue. The patient must replace lost fluids, preferably by drinking fluids rather than intravenous administration. The patient should be encouraged to drink regularly since thirst is not a reliable indicator.
Pain.	Pain might result from involvement of central nervous system infections; peripheral neuropathy; patient immobility; malignant or infectious processes in the body; or from labored breathing. Standard pain management is suggested, namely pain medication, relaxation techniques, massage.
Patient Education.	Patients have complained of being overwhelmed with information. Others have suffered great mental anguish because accurate information was withheld. In general, the manner of presentation is very important. Education must proceed at a rate the patient is able to absorb and in terms and language the patient understands.
Patient-Nurse Interaction.	Certain themes common to AIDS patients are shared by patients suffering from other terminal illnesses. For example, terminally ill patients greatly value their relationships with their nurses. The patient-nurse relationship is very sensitive—having both positive and negative potential. On the positive side, the nurse makes the patient experience less lonely and less traumatic, physically and mentally. On the negative side, the nurse can reinforce or trigger negative self-image, such as guilt over being sexually active, a homosexual, or a drug-user, or having infected a sexual partner. With cancer patients, when nurses lose hope so do their patients, who become more likely to pursue "quack" treatments. A difficult or angry patient should be met with calm reassurance. Many AIDS patients fear abandonment. Calmly reassure them that quality care will continue.

Physiotherapy.	Exercise of AIDS patients has often been neglected; occupational therapists have not even been notified. Particularly now that drug and other regimens provide some hope of slowing disease progression and lessening the symptoms and conditions of AIDS, exercise may have some therapeutic benefit and make the patient more comfortable.
	Coughing and deep breathing exercises should be introduced early into treatment. If pneumonia is present, pursed-lip breathing should be taught. Speech, physical and occupational therapies may be necessary to improve function or to relearn skills following central nervous system infection.
Sensitivity.	While protective equipment shields the health care worker from pathogens, the health care worker need not be insensitive to the patient's needs for human contact. Masks hide a person's face, but need not hide a person's warmth or personality. Interact with the patient as a human being, not solely as a source of infection.
Skin.	Skin care is particularly necessary as bedsores are often aggravated by herpes viruses. Care involves frequent inspection of the skin, and shifting of the patient position every two hours. Ointments may be prescribed; instruct patient in proper use.

from other patients. However, HIV-infected persons should not be barred from other areas of the hospital as long as they are physically and mentally capable of maintaining infection control. Actively coughing patients should wear masks when out of their rooms.

In some instances AIDS patients have been isolated because of the adverse psychological effect they have on other patients. The solution to this difficult problem may lie in educational efforts aimed at the general public. In some larger urban hospitals AIDS patients have been housed together in a separate ward, not to isolate them, but to better concentrate the special skills needed for their care through corps of volunteer health care workers.

Incidents of HIV Transmission

A number of documented cases exist of HIV transmission to health care workers through contaminated substances from AIDS patients. Reportedly, HIV has been transmitted to health care workers by needlestick accidents, mucous membrane exposure, and possibly skin exposure to contaminated substances.

HIV is not highly contagious. In the majority of accidental exposures, HIV transmission has not occurred. In some instances, health care workers have caught other diseases, such as hepatitis B and *Cryptococcus,* from AIDS patients without contracting HIV.

Needlestick accidents, a very common occurrence, account for the majority of accidental exposures to HIV-contaminated substances. In one study of over 900 accidental exposures to HIV, approximately 75 percent were needlestick accidents. Approximately 85 percent of the time, blood or blood serum was the contaminated substance involved.

In the several documented cases of HIV transmission occurring from needlestick accidents, transmission occurred from both deep and superficial punctures. The contaminated substance in the needles was usually blood; in one case fluid containing blood from membranes surrounding the lungs was the substance.

One health care worker had blood splatter across her face and into her mouth when working with a vacuum tube that popped open. She was wearing glasses and did not think any blood had entered her eyes. She had facial acne but no open wounds. She washed immediately after exposure. She was seronegative upon testing 8 weeks later, but seropositive when she attempted to donate blood 9 months later.

Two health care workers apparently contracted HIV from blood exposures to broken skin in separate incidents. One, during a cardiac arrest incident had a small amount of blood on her index finger for about 20 minutes; she also had chapped hands. Another worker was involved in a major blood spill, in which blood covered most of her hands and forearms. She was not wearing gloves, but washed several minutes after exposure. She had dermatitis on one ear and may have touched it. In dermatitis, the skin is itching and red, and small lesions may develop.

HIV may have been transmitted by feces in a couple of situations. In one instance, a mother was infected by her infant. In the report published by the

CDC, the mother, who was participating in the child's care, reported no needlestick accidents, but frequently exposed her hands to feces, blood, saliva, and nasal secretions. She seldom wore gloves and was careless about hand-washing after exposure. In another suspected case, an English woman working in a nursing home may have contracted HIV from a man who was diagnosed some time after his death as having AIDS. The woman's hands were frequently exposed for prolonged periods to the man's feces and other body substances.

These few instances document that HIV transmission can occur through accidental exposure. However, out of hundreds of such exposures involving HIV-contaminated substances, HIV transmission has occurred in only a few cases. Most exposures occurred because safety procedures were not followed. Better procedures and, no doubt, safer equipment will be developed because of AIDS. With careful adherence to safety procedures and a bit of forethought, the risk of contracting HIV in the medical setting can be eliminated entirely.

Needlestick Prevention

An estimated 200 needlestick accidents occur each year in larger urban medical centers. A large number of these still go unreported. Many health care workers disregard proper procedures for needle handling and in-house–accident reporting regulations.

The cause of most needlestick accidents are, in order of *decreasing* frequency: (1) recapping of needles, (2) improper disposal of needles or sharp objects, and (3) improper operation of needle-cutting devices. All situations are easy to avoid.

According to CDC recommendations needles should not be capped, bent, or removed from disposable syringes, or otherwise manipulated by hand. In many urban centers nurses now use forceps to handle needles and needle caps and sheaths.

A needle need not be recapped, resheathed, or cut from the syringe before being discarded. Forceps can be used to take the needle off the syringe and place it directly in a disposal container. Needle disposal boxes must be collected often enough to avoid overfilling.

If forceps are not available, it is suggested that a needle be recapped by placing the sheath on a level surface, inserting the tip of the needle into the sheath, and then tilting the needle and sheath vertically until the sheath slides down, covering the needle. Alternatively, caps with 1- to 2-centimeter diameter, funnel-shaped shields have been shown to be effective at decreasing the number of accidental misses in a recapping trial. Manufacturers may soon be responding to the need for needlestick prevention.

One should never hold the needle in one hand and the sheath in the other and try to bring them together horizontally. Reportedly, this technique results in the most needlestick accidents.

Since familiarity can lead to a lack of caution, aggressive and continuing educational efforts must be made so that health care workers continue to adhere to proper procedures.

Handwashing

Handwashing may be the single most important procedure for preventing infection in the hospital. Hands can transmit disease-causing organisms from an infected patient to another patient or a health care worker. handwashing is defined as the vigorous, brief rubbing together of all surfaces of lathered hands, followed by rinsing under a stream of water. No one knows how long to rub the hands together; 10 seconds is considered minimum.

Human skin has a number of resident bacteria that are not very virulent unless they are introduced deep into the body. The mechanical removal of external germs is accomplished by washing hands with plain soaps or detergents. For surgery and invasive procedures, germs are chemically removed with antimicrobial agents that kill germs or inhibit their growth.

Compliance is a major issue with handwashing. Handwashing is an inconvenience when workers are busy, as they commonly are; frequent handwashing often causes chapped hands; and workers may not be in the habit of washing hands. Constant reinforcement of the requirement is necessary, focusing either on the benefits of handwashing or the avoidance of risk.

Sinks should be located in convenient areas with handwashing accessories and paper towels. The sinks should be designed so as to minimize splash and recontamination, for example, with foot pedals, or handles that can be manipulated with the elbows. Soap should be left on racks so it will drain. Liquid soap containers should be well cleaned between refills.

Protective Equipment Use

Gloves. Gloves are very important for the health of both the patient and the health care worker. The hands frequently have lesions which penetrate the outer layer of skin. Such lesions may not be visible to the eye but may serve as sites of infection or transmission. Lesions often exist near the fingernails, which is also where blood or other substances can become impacted. In one study, blood remained under the fingernails of dentists for up to 5 days, presenting a risk to the dentist, the patients, and the dentist's family.

For suggested use of *sterile gloves,* see Figure 27.

Nonsterile gloves are generally worn to prevent gross microbiological contamination of hands. Nonsterile gloves should be used when handling blood or body fluids and tissues, when handling objects contaminated by these substances, and when cleaning contaminated surfaces.

Handwashing should follow glove use. Gloves are used to prevent gross contamination. Gloves are not perfect barriers and may develop tiny perforations, allowing contamination of the hands. Also, bacteria multiply rapidly on gloved hands, which provide a warm environment with plenty of moisture.

Bandages. Contamination of open wounds with contaminated substances is very common among health care workers, ranking with needlestick accidents as a major cause of accidental exposure. In order to protect both themselves and the patient, health care workers should cover any open wounds with waterproof bandages.

Figure 26: Handwashing Indications

Handwashing depends on the type, intensity, duration and sequence of activity. Good handwashing should remove all organisms from the skin that do not belong on the body.

Handwashing Suggested

- Before care of immunocompromised patient.
- After caring for a patient infected by virulent micro-organisms.
- Before switching from one care site to another on the same patient.
- Before and after touching wounds.
- Before and after invasive procedures.
- After prolonged and intense contact with a patient.
- After touching potentially contaminated objects.
- After touching visibly soiled objects.
- After wearing gloves.
- Immediately after contact of naked hands with blood, body fluids, tissues, feces, urine, saliva, nasal secretions, contaminated dressings, etc.
- Between patients.
- When in doubt.

Handwashing Not Suggested

- After superficial contact with patient.
- After touching an object not visibly soiled.
- After taking blood pressure.

Gowns. It is recommended that reusable or disposable gowns be worn when clothing is likely to be exposed to blood or other body fluids and substances. Any person involved in cleaning or sterilizing equipment should wear gowns and heavy-duty rubber gloves.

It is debatable whether clothing can transmit disease to and from the patient. Some common bacteria can be transmitted from health care workers' clothing to patients' clothing, but whether this poses any threat of infection remains to be proved. Some infection control specialists suggest that lightweight, disposable gowns be worn when attending an immunocompromised patient. Some infection control practitioners suggest changing uniforms daily.

Masks and Shields. It is recommended that masks be worn when a patient is actively coughing, has diagnosed tuberculosis, or when the diagnosis of tuberculosis has not been ruled out. Masks are not considered necessary when attending an alert patient who is not coughing.

Protective eyewear, in the form of goggles or chin-length shields, should be worn when splashing, splattering, or aerosols, airborne droplets, of blood or body fluids or substances can occur. In some situations, face shields may be desirable whenever handling contaminated substances.

Cleaning Activities

Any health care workers performing the following procedures should wear gowns, face shields if necessary, and heavy-duty rubber gloves. Gloves should be inspected frequently, as many chemicals adversely affect or penetrate rubber. Skin contact with cleaning fluids and contaminated substances should be avoided.

Sterilization is the destruction of all forms of microbial life, including viruses and bacterial spores. A suggested listing of the various techniques, in order of preference, is (1) steam under pressure and autoclaves, (2) prolonged dry heat, (3) ethylene oxide gas, and (4) boiling water. Ten minutes should kill HIV, but Bacillus spores, a bacterium, may survive for hours. Autoclaves are considered the cheapest method of sterilization. All apparatus used for sterilization should be checked weekly for contamination.

Disinfection is the general term for the cleaning of objects that cannot be sterilized, such as heat-sensitive objects or objects too large to fit into sterilizing apparatus. Disinfection is alternatively defined as an intermediate step between sterilization and cleaning. Disinfection is sometimes improperly called "cold sterilization," but disinfection is not sterilization.

Disinfection is usually performed with liquid chemicals. The object is immersed in the chemicals, or the chemicals are spread over the object, as when disinfecting a countertop. When an object is immersed in a fluid, some agitation is usually required to dislodge air bubbles. The object must be exposed to the chemical for 10 to 20 minutes according to manufacturer's specifications.

Cleaning removes germs rather than kills them. Both disinfection and cleaning attempt to reduce the number of germs, making them less of a threat to a person should exposure occur.

Effectiveness of Cleaning. The effectiveness of a cleaning activity depends on several factors: (1) the *concentration* of the chemical in the cleaning solution, (2) the length of *time* the germ is exposed to the chemicals, (3) the *temperature* during exposure, and (4) the *protective effect* of any other *substances surrounding the germ.* In general the higher the concentration or the higher the temperature, the shorter the contact time needed. However, blood, body tissues, or dirt may in some instances quickly neutralize chemicals, sometimes before the chemical can effectively destroy the germs. Thus, if a pathogen is protected by other substances, then larger volumes of cleaning solutions are needed. Care should be taken that any dried substances become thoroughly soaked with cleaning solution. Ideally, dried substances should become suspended in the solution. Be sure that exposure time is adequate.

Sometimes, organic material can shield a virus from the disinfecting chemicals, so the physical removal of organic material may be important in any cleaning activity. If an object is heavily contaminated, some infection control specialists suggest autoclaving the object first, then physically removing the organic matter, and then following with another sterilization of the cleaned surfaces.

Figure 27: Suggested Sterile Glove Use

Wear sterile gloves when:

- Touching any non-intact skin.
- Touching any mucous membrane.
- Touching the anal or genital region.
- Dressing or changing wounds.
- Drawing blood.
- Performing any invasive procedures.

Change sterile gloves when:

- Changing patients (and handwash).
- Switching care site or activity on same patient (and handwash).

Remove gloves:

- Before leaving the caregiving area (and handwash).

Do Not:

- Reuse gloves.

Patient Care Equipment

Patient care equipment is generally divided into three groups according to cleaning needs: critical, semicritical, and noncritical.

Critical equipment must be sterilized, because this equipment is used for invasive techniques. It is inserted directly into the bloodstream or other normally sterile areas of the body. Examples of critical care items are hypodermic needles, scalpels, cardiac catheters, blood compartments of hemodialyzers, implants, and certain components of heart-lung machines.

Semicritical equipment frequently comes into contact with mucous membranes, but does not ordinarily penetrate them or other body surfaces. If possible, semicritical equipment should be sterilized. Otherwise, meticulous cleaning followed by appropriate application of high-level disinfectants is performed. Examples of semicritical equipment are endoscopes, endotracheal tubes, and noninvasive fiberoptic equipment.

Noncritical equipment includes items which either do not touch the patient or touch only intact skin, such as bedboards, blood-pressure cuffs, crutches, etc. Unless such equipment is visibly soiled with blood or other body substances, only cleaning is required.

HIV Inactivation

HIV Survival. HIV reportedly can survive in a solution of fetal calf blood diluted to 10 percent (1 part blood, 9 parts neutral fluid) for 14 days at room temperature (22 to 25°C) and up to 11 days at 100°F (37°C).

Dried HIV was found to lose approximately 90 to 99 percent of its infectivity after a matter of hours at room temperature. Complete inactivity of dried viruses required 3 days at room temperature. These experiments were conducted with extremely high concentrations of virus, higher than found in biological systems. Some blood products and commercial clotting factors are dried, and evidently HIV survives this drying as well, since these products reportedly transmit HIV.

Methods of Inactivation. *Heat* can inactivate HIV in blood solutions. A 10 percent solution of human serum heated to 130°F (56°C) showed no detectable levels of HIV in 10 minutes. In a 90 percent solution of human serum, HIV was inactivated in 30 minutes at 130°F (56°C), and in 60 minutes at 100°F (37°C). Freeze-dried blood required slightly higher temperatures for the same time of exposure. A quite different length of HIV survival was reported in fetal calf blood as noted above.

Survival times of dry HIV, when exposed to heat, might be different. Heat-treated FVIII factor has transmitted HIV infection, although heat treatment greatly reduces the risk.

Radiation is an experimental form of HIV inactivation. HIV is reportedly sensitive to both gamma rays and ultraviolet light. Radiation is currently not considered a good way to inactivate HIV, since radiation, if it does not kill an organism, can cause mutations.

Use of *chemicals* present in many commercial cleaning agents is the best way for most people to inactivate HIV.

Tested Soaps and Detergents. In general, any soap, detergent, and chemical effective against hepatitis B should be effective against HIV. A number of commercial cleaning agents which have proved effective in inactivating HIV are mentioned below. For these tests HIV was cultured in fetal calf serum. In culture, HIV was exposed to the cleaning agents for 2 to 10 minutes at room temperature (21 to 25°C).

When disinfecting objects, one should remember the factors of temperature, length of exposure, chemical concentration, and the protective effect of any other substances present. People should wear gloves when handling chemicals or performing cleaning activity.

Bleach is the preferred cleaning agent of many laboratories for cleaning counters, floors, etc. However, dirt quickly neutralizes the active ingredient in bleach. A 10 percent bleach solution is generally used. A 1 percent solution was found to inactivate HIV. Bleach is inexpensive. If more disinfecting activity is needed, more bleach should be added. Unfortunately, bleach corrodes almost everything, including most plastics and metal. Thus, bleach is not suitable for many medical applications. Bleach is very toxic to any living tissue; it can cause burns when spilled on human skin.

Ethanol (grain alcohol) in a 50 percent solution inactivates HIV; 95 percent solutions are commercially available. Ethanol should be used with care, since blood and protein tissues seem to rapidly neutralize its effects.

Isopropyl alcohol (rubbing alcohol) in a 35 percent solution is also effective. Drugstore alcohol is frequently 70 percent; read the label to determine the percentage.

Lysol and *Nonidet P-40* inactivate HIV, Lysol at 0.5 percent solution (commercially available at 3 percent), and Nonidet P-40 at 1 percent soluton. *Paraformaldehydes* and *phenols* are also effective. The cleaning agent Tween-20 was not effective. Formalin (2%) was effective, but too slow.

Other Infection Control Issues

Exposure to Human Skin. If an open wound is exposed to HIV-contaminated substances, it should be immediately washed out with large amounts of hydrogen peroxide or a 10 percent solution of bleach.

If healthy skin is exposed to contaminated substances, immediately wash the exposed area with a 70 percent solution of ethanol (grain alcohol), or isopropyl (rubbing) alcohol, or a 3 percent solution of hydrogen peroxide.

If mucous membranes (eyes, mouth, etc.) are exposed to a contaminated substance, immediately flush with large amounts of water.

Blood Spills. Any person touching a spill of blood or other body substances, such as vomit, urine, or feces should wear gloves. Using a 10 percent or stronger bleach solution, the person should surround the spill with bleach, then work inward toward the substance with a mop, working slowly and carefully to avoid splashing or aerosols. Protective face gear and gowns should be worn when cleaning up major spills. With larger spills, the blood should be removed with towels (which should then be properly disposed of or placed in a bucket of bleach solution), before the floor is mopped. It is important to remember that organic materials and dirt can neutralize the bleach and that exposure time must be sufficient, usually 10 minutes maximum. Mop heads should be soaked in bleach solution after cleaning spills.

Infective Waste. Any object that is contaminated with blood or other body substances may be considered potentially infectious. It is not practical, however, to treat all waste as infectious waste.

Special precautions should be taken with microbiological specimens, pathology waste, blood specimens and blood products, contaminated dressings, and disposable equipment.

It is recommended that disposable infectious waste, such as contaminated bandages, dressings, tubing, etc., be placed in color-coded waterproof bags. Another method of labeling is the designation "H/A precautions" (hepatitis/AIDS) or "Blood/Body-Fluid precautions." The necessary staff should be told what labeling designation is being used. Labeling is an area where confidentiality can easily be lost, and thus there is a need to stress confidentiality with all employees. Some references recommend double-bagging infectious waste, while others feel double-bagging is unnecessary unless the exterior of the bag is visibly contaminated. In England, incineration is the preferred method of disposing of infectious waste.

Needles and other sharp objects should be placed in puncture-resistant containers, such as plastic bottles with screw-on caps.

Proper handling of infective waste is an issue of importance both to the health care worker and the community. The media have reported that young children have been found playing with HIV-contaminated blood vials and HIV-contaminated hypodermic needles improperly disposed of in a waste bin.

Housekeeping. Housekeeping staffs need to be educated in HIV transmission, epidemiology, and waste labeling techniques. They should be given specific and exact instructions on how to act, what to touch, and what to avoid. Written materials should be provided.

Laundry. Visibly contaminated linens and clothes should be transported in hot-water-soluble bags (which dissolve in hot water) so they can be thrown directly into the wash without further human contact. Again, double-bagging of contaminated clothes and linen is not suggested unless the outside of the bag is visibly soiled.

It is generally agreed that standard hospital laundry equipment, using a normal laundry cycle is sufficient; wash water should be over 140°F (60 to 70°C) with normal amount of bleach; drying temperatures should be over 212°F (100°C).

Some hospitals presoak all their laundry in bleach solutions before washing. The CDC does not recommend presoaking, but it may be wise if bedding or clothing is heavily contaminated with blood or other infectious substances.

Dishes. Dishes and eating utensils of AIDS patients should be handled with ordinary hospital precautions. If they are visibly soiled with blood or other body fluids or substances, they should be cleaned or soaked in bleach solution before being taken to the kitchen. Gloves should be worn when hand-washing dishes which are contaminated with blood or body substances.

In nonhospital settings dishes can be washed in hot soapy water.

Administrative Concerns

Degree of Risk. AIDS is not yet common in all geographical regions. Years will pass before many rural hospitals will see AIDS patients. Experts generally agree that routine HIV testing of all hospital patients is not necessary. However, some debate exists whether AIDS-style precautions are necessary for handling every patient, blood specimen, tissue specimen, and bag of infectious waste. There is also disagreement whether contaminated blood and other substances or the beds of AIDS patients should be marked. Any labeling is likely to destroy confidentiality.

Some public health officials suggest that hospitals must decide on a local level how to react to the AIDS epidemic. Since AIDS will probably spread throughout the United States and the world, concentrated in high-risk groups but gradually affecting all types of individuals, all hospitals should have established policies to deal with the epidemic.

An urban hospital which sees many AIDS cases might not label AIDS patients or their substances, instead preferring to maintain a level of infection control which treats all patients as potentially infectious. Rural hospitals may wish to individually label AIDS patients and their contaminated substances, since a blanket approach to using hepatitis and AIDS precautions would be unnecessary and could lead to noncompliance.

Infected Employees. By most current recommendations, HIV-infected employees without symptoms should not be restricted from employment. Health care workers who are immunosuppressed should be excused from attending any potentially infectious patient. Restrictions or special precautions discussed here relate to health care workers who perform invasive procedures. An indication of the risk involved appears in the study reporting transmission of hepatitis B from surgeon to patient estimated at 1 in 1 million per year in Great Britain, occurring in clusters where one surgeon infects several patients.

Health care workers (HIV-infected or not) with acute diarrhea, oral or facial herpes lesions, herpes zoster, weeping dermatitis or leaking lesions which cannot be properly covered, or infectious respiratory ailments should refrain from patient care and the handling of patient-care equipment until the condition resolves. In general, any illness which reduces the mental or physical ability of the health care worker may necessitate excluding the health care worker from specific tasks. It is suggested that the status of an HIV-infected health care worker be determined on a case-by-case basis.

Confidentiality is a major concern; news travels fast among staff, and the community may pressure for dismissal of the infected employee.

Pregnant Health Care Workers. Recommendations vary concerning pregnant health care workers. As long as infection control procedures are followed, little risk of HIV transmission exists. Concerned individuals suggest that pregnant health care workers be excluded from caring for AIDS patients since cytomegalovirus, Epstein-Barr virus, and some herpes viruses can cause fetal infection, and these infections are often present in AIDS patients.

Employee Exposure to HIV. Employees should immediately report all accidents and exposures, including needlesticks, cuts and lacerations, exposures of lesions or mucous membranes, prolonged skin exposure, etc., to the designated persons.

If a health care worker has been exposed to a potentially contaminated substance, then the Centers for Disease Control (CDC) and the American Hospital Association (AHA) recommend that the patient be requested to give consent for HIV testing. If the patient is seropositive, or refuses to give consent, the health care worker is requested to give consent for testing. Ideally, the health care worker should have a baseline test immediately, then be tested every 3 months for 1 year. The exposed employee should be instructed in the prevention of HIV transmission.

Patient Exposure to HIV. In a situation where a health care worker bleeds into a patient during surgery, the health care worker should be clinically assessed to determine the likelihood of infection. If this evaluation suggests that the health care worker is at high risk for infection, then the worker should be asked to consent to an AIDS test. If the health care worker tests positive, then the exposed patient should be informed and offered testing and counseling. If the health care worker tests negative, then subsequent tests should be taken at 3-month intervals for at least 1 year. Contact with the patient should be maintained.

Staff Protection. Hospital administration is under some legal obligation to provide employees with the proper equipment, education, policies, and procedures to enable employees to work safely. These obligations may vary by city, county, and state.

Administration should seriously consider the situation of an employee who might become infected at work. Before an incident occurs, plans should be made for insurance or proper coverage for loss of earnings and for possible retraining and reemployment elsewhere.

Employers have an obligation to create an apparatus for discussing health and safety issues and allowing feedback from front-line employees on policies, procedures, equipment, etc.

It is suggested that health care workers have regular physical examinations, be immunized with the hepatitis B vaccine, develop the habit of making careful note of their illness patterns or changes in normal body functions, and have periodic laboratory evaluations.

Noncompliance. The lack of compliance with infection control procedures is a problem. Compliance might be improved through monitoring, continuing educational reinforcement, and peer pressure.

Lack of compliance can stem from obstacles to procedure such as inconveniently located sinks, lack of cleaning supplies, unacceptable cleaning products, and understaffing. Lack of compliance can also result from lack of knowledge or lack of appreciation for the importance of the procedure. Staff feedback is necessary for solving compliance problems.

Areas of Special Concern

Hemodialysis. To date, there have been no documented cases of HIV transmission in the hemodialysis setting. Reports exist of hepatitis B transmission and delta factor transmission (a cofactor in developing life-threatening hepatitis) between hospitalized patients in the hemodialysis setting because of extensive contamination of the environment due to blood accidents or contamination of instruments.

The CDC does not recommend isolation of the HIV-infected hemodialysis patient. However, one report suggests that delta-positive patients be hemodialyzed separately from delta-negative patients.

Seropositive patients should be able to be dialyzed in either freestanding or hospital-based units. Recommendations point to careful health care worker adherence to standard blood-related infection control precautions: appropriate decontamination of equipment and surfaces; and restriction of nondisposable equipment to one patient only, unless sterilization occurs between uses. Some practitioners recommend that the dialyzer, along with the blood lines, be discarded after use and that the dialyzer not be used for more than one patient.

It has been suggested that hemodialysis patients who have received multiple blood transfusions be screened for HIV.

Obstetrics. Blood and body fluid precautions should be followed for both mother and baby during birth. Gloves, gowns, goggles, and masks or face shields should be worn during birthing, while handling the placenta, the infant, blood, or amniotic fluid, and until all instruments and surfaces are decontaminated or disposed of.

Both antepartum (before birth) and postpartum (after birth) women should be able to share toilet facilities with others. An HIV-infected father poses little risk to the infant unless he is actively infected with other transmissible diseases.

Laboratory. In the laboratory all specimens of semen, blood, saliva, tears, urine, cerebrospinal fluid, and brain tissue from infected humans or primates are considered potentially infectious. Gloves and gowns should be worn when handling these fluids and tissues.

Strict handwashing procedures are recommended after handling contaminated materials, after completing experiments, and before leaving the laboratory. Cuts and abrasions should be covered properly. Mouth-pipetting is, of course, prohibited, as are eating, drinking, food or beverage storage, smoking, and fingernail-biting. All equipment which could generate spills or aerosols should be covered with disposable material such as aluminum foil. All surfaces should be kept clean.

The staff should be well versed in emergency decontamination procedures for blood spills and contaminated surfaces.

Public access to the laboratory should be restricted. Work should proceed with the doors closed.

Any experiments on human serum or infectious sources should be conducted with federal guidelines for Biological Safety Level 2 practices. Any culturing on a research laboratory scale is conducted with Level 2 practices and with containment equipment of Biological Safety Level 3.

Contaminated glassware, equipment, materials, and wastes should be decontaminated before being washed or discarded. Laboratory clothing should be decontaminated before being laundered or discarded.

It is suggested that baseline blood samples be drawn from all laboratory workers.

Emergency Personnel. Paramedics, emergency medical technicians, law enforcement personnel, lifeguards, medical care personnel, and any other individuals who may have to provide emergency health care should be well versed in the facts of HIV transmission and prevention.

In the hospital or health care setting, plastic airways constructed for mouth-to-mouth resuscitation should be placed both in accessible areas and next to beds of high-risk patients. In emergency rooms, easy access to gowns, gloves, and goggles should be arranged.

Blood precautions are suggested for all patients for whom no medical history is available. The risk of HIV transmission varies by region. In a San Francisco study 18 percent of 121 men and women who died unexpectedly were seropositive and had no pathological or laboratory signs of HIV infection.

Dentistry. HIV patients can be safely handled in the dental office as long as some preparations are made in advance. The major concern is that certain surfaces can become contaminated, because they cannot be sterilized. Thus some work surfaces, light switch handles, instrument trays, brackets, chair arms, sink faucet handles, shade guides, and other surfaces which may be contaminated by aerosols or splatterings should be covered with disposable material. Plastic and aluminum foil have been suggested for this purpose. Gloves should be worn during disposal of such coverings.

Goggles, masks, gloves, and gowns are generally recommended for surgi-

Figure 28: Hygiene in the Home

Personal:	A person should wash his or her hands after coming into contact with their own semen, vaginal fluids, mucous, or blood. For the HIV-infected person, frequent handwashing is a good idea; the hands bring germs to the mouth. Use soft toothbrush to clean under fingernails. Do not wash to excess. Individuals should wash their hands before preparing food. A sneezing or coughing individual should cover his or her mouth with a handkerchief, tissue, or mask. Inflamed skin, minor cuts, open or "weeping" (moist) skin wounds should be covered with waterproof or other suitable dressings. Body fluids can be flushed down the toilet. If the plumbing systems accept them, tampons and condoms can be flushed down the toilet.
Kitchen:	An AIDS patient can safely cook for others. He or she should wash hands before handling food. Normal sanitary practices should be followed. Don't lick fingers or spoon while preparing food. Kitchen surfaces should be cleaned with scouring powder to remove food particles. The inside of refrigerators should be cleaned with soap and water to control molds, bleach is not considered necessary. The kitchen floor should be mopped weekly, food spills should be cleaned up as they occur. Mop water should not be poured down the sink where food is prepared. Do not use dirty-looking sponges to clean dishes. Use separate sponges to clean kitchen and bathroom.
Bathroom:	Toothbrushes should not be shared. Towels and washclothes should not be shared without laundering. Mop the floor at least once weekly with a solution containing bleach. Bleach solutions should be used to clean up spills of blood, urine, feces, etc. Mop water should not be poured down sink where food is prepared. A container of bleach solution, changed daily, can be a receptacle for tampons, razors, dental floss, or anything that is exposed to body fluids. Sponges used to clean up spills of body substances on the floor should not be used in the kitchen.
Mops/Sponges:	Mops and sponges used to clean up the floor or contaminated substances can be soaked in a bleach solution. Mops should be agitated so the bleach gets into all parts of the mophead.
Bleach:	Bleach is a very strong chemical agent (oxidizer). Flush drains before and after use. Keep area well ventilated. *DO NOT mix bleach with other household or commercial cleaners* such as toilet bowl cleaners, rust removers, acid or ammonia containing products. If bleach is mixed with these substances, deadly gases may be chemically released.
Dishes:	Dishes may be shared. Wash in hot soapy water, rinse in hot water, and dry. Some infection control specialists suggest letting dishes soak and that the water should be hot enough to require gloves. Disinfectants are not considered necessary. If the dishes are visibly contaminated with blood or body fluids, soak first in a bleach solution.

Laundry:	Clothes visibly soiled with blood or other body substances should be handled with gloves, placed into water-soluble bags (available at hospital supply stores) which can be thrown into the washing machine without further human contact. Such clothes might be pre-soaked in a bleach solution before washing. Otherwise sufficient bleach can be added to the washing machine. Water temperature should be 60 to 70 degrees Centigrade. Dryers should have a temperature of 100 degrees Centigrade or higher.
Animals:	While animals offer emotional support, there is a conflict between benefit and risk for the patient. Animals carry a risk for the HIV-infected person. For example, cats carry toxoplasmosis which is excreted in their feces. Petting or handling the pet usually does not transmit this parasite; an individual has to ingest the parasite's eggs. HIV-infected individuals, ideally, should not handle cat boxes; if necessary they should do so only while wearing gloves and masks. Handwash afterwards. Cat boxes should be handled gently, keeping airborne dust to a minimum. Litter boxes should be changed daily, ridding them of toxoplasmosis eggs. Cats must be kept off surfaces where food is prepared. Ticks and fleas carry toxoplasmosis. Don't let animals eat raw meat or prey; they can contract parasites from their prey. If possible, restrict the animal from contact with other animals. If gardening in potentially contaminated soil, wear gloves. Fish tanks and bird cages also present problems. HIV-infected people should not clean or handle these items. Dogs can carry parasitic worms and are suspected of sharing respiratory diseases with humans.
Children:	Children frequently pick up infections from school or daycare and bring them home, such as cytomegalovirus, herpes zoster (chickenpox), and intestinal parasites. Children might also play in parasite-contaminated dirt and/or sandboxes, if these sites are frequented by animals. An HIV-infected person might wish to avoid contact with the secretions of children.
Diet:	Unpasteurized milk and milk products should be avoided by HIV-infected individuals; they are associated with Salmonella bacteria infections.
Infective Waste:	Anything soiled with blood or body substances, such as underpants, bandages and dressings, and medical gloves, should be considered infective waste and disposed of in durable plastic bags. Some infection control experts suggest double-bagging while others say double-bagging is necessary only when the exterior of the first bag is visibly soiled. Needles and sharp instruments should be placed into puncture- resistant containers, such as plastic bottles with screw-on tops, before disposal. British health authorities recommend incineration of infective waste. In the U.S., disposal according to local solid fill regulations is suggested by CDC. Dispose in a manner such that animals, children, and the homeless are not endangered.

Figure 28: Hygiene in the Home (Continued)

Ventilation:	Keep living areas well ventilated. Airborne diseases are less infectious when diluted by air.
Organic Food:	Food grown in human or animal waste should be washed before use. Fruits should be peeled.
Exposure to Human Skin:	If an open wound is exposed to HIV contaminated substances, immediately wash it out with large amounts of hydrogen peroxide (3 percent in water–read the label) or a 10 percent solution of bleach. If healthy skin is exposed to contaminated substances, immediately wash the exposed area with a 70 percent solution of ethanol (ethyl or grain alcohol), or isopropyl (rubbing) alcohol, or a 3 percent solution of hydrogen peroxide. If a mucous membrane (eyes, mouth) is exposed to a contaminated substance, immediately flush it with large amounts of water.
Blood Spills:	Wear gloves when cleaning up blood spills, vomit, or other spills of body substances. Wear aprons for cleaning up large spills. Surround the spill with bleach and slowly work in to avoid splashes and airborne droplets. Towels may be needed to clean up gross contamination before cleaning with bleach solution. Discard these towels as infective waste or soak in a bleach solution.

cal procedures when blood is likely to be encountered or when aerosols are freely generated. Glove use is generally recommended for all contact with mucous membranes. Routine testing of all dental patients is not recommended.

Home Care. Home care for HIV-infected people is often a desirable course of action. Patients may stay at home between bouts of hospitalization, but must be physically and emotionally stable before being considered for home care. Home care allows patients a degree of autonomy, which enhances their mental and, perhaps, physical status. Home care also greatly reduces the cost of treatment. In addition, home care may allow for some reconciliation between AIDS patients and their families and friends before their deaths. Finally, it may allow terminally ill patients to die more peacefully among familiar surroundings.

Before home care can be considered, the family or caring group must be assessed on the basis of their ability to care for the patient and to adhere to infection control procedures which protect the patient, themselves, and their community. The family's commitment to care must be assessed, particularly if the patient and family have been estranged. The family should be directed to community resources for counseling or to family bereavement support groups.

If possible, a health care worker or other knowledgeable person should visit the home to check for conditions such as poor hygiene or likelihood of exposure to illnesses such as respiratory or childhood diseases which may lead to the patient's development of opportunistic infections.

Family members or caregivers should be educated in HIV transmission, epidemiology, prevention, and infection control procedures. Caregivers should be instructed in the importance of handwashing. They should also be taught to monitor the patient for respiratory complications, fever, change in amount or appearance of sputum or bowel activity, and changes in cognitive functions or behaviors. Caregivers should watch for shortness of breath and indications of cyanosis (turning blue from lack of oxygen). Instruction in use of oxygen equipment may also be necessary.

With seropositive children, careful attention must be given to monitoring growth, development, and cognitive functions. In infants, parents must watch for crying and postural or behavioral symptoms of pain. Caregivers should wear gloves when changing diapers. Afterward, they should wash the rectal area well with mild soap and water and apply a thin ointment or petroleum jelly, watchful for the development of lesions.

The AIDS patient can share the bathroom with other family members as long as infection control procedures are observed. Any area visibly soiled by the patient should be cleaned with bleach. A container of bleach solution can be placed under the sink for discarding dressings, razors, or other small potentially contaminated instruments. The bleach solution in the container should be changed daily.

For home disposal of infectious waste, the CDC recommends that blood and other body fluids be flushed down the toilet, that spills be cleaned with bleach solution, and that items contaminated with blood or body fluids be placed in an impervious and sturdy plastic bag which in turn is placed inside a second bag and disposed of according to local solid-waste regulations. Note, however, that the British equivalent of the CDC suggests that such wastes be incinerated since animals and homeless people often rip waste bags open to inspect the contents.

For hypodermic syringes and needles, full-strength bleach can be drawn into them before needle destruction and disposal within a puncture-resistant container such as a plastic jar with a screw-on cap.

20. Volunteering

The AIDS epidemic may be outrunning the efforts of public health and education officials, shackled as they are by monetary limitations. An effective response to the AIDS epidemic will require efforts from many members of the private sector; otherwise, the facilities of many major medical centers or cities may be overwhelmed. Although AIDS will probably continue to be concentrated in certain regions, its effects will be widespread, encompassing the social circles of virtually all human beings.

Help is needed in every aspect of anti-AIDS efforts. In most larger cities existing AIDS-service organizations tend to be coordinators of volunteer efforts. These service organizations utilize volunteers in education activities, office help, promotion efforts, and patient care. The need for patient care is the greatest, for both emotional and financial reasons. The initial cases of AIDS cost almost $140,000 each, because patients, evicted from their homes or with no one to care for them, stayed in the hospital between bouts of serious illness. Home care is less costly and, in most cases, more pleasant, but requires volunteer support.

Suggested volunteer roles, according to the Gay Men's Health Crisis in New York City, include: (1) the *ombudsman*, who documents complaints from the patient regarding social or medical mistreatment, resolves problems, performs investigations, and confronts the medical or legal authorities when fault is found; (2) *buddies*, who are assigned to one patient at a time and act as a friend, providing transportation, cooking meals, cleaning house, and doing laundry; (3) the *support manager*, a highly trained person who visits the patient, discusses difficult psychological issues, and describes options of care and support; (4) the *intake volunteer*, who visits the patient in the hospital within a day or two and assesses individual needs for support; (5) the *resource manager*, who handles the complicated forms required for insurance, disability, and social security, overwhelming tasks for the emotionally and physically taxed patient; (6) the *legal advocate*, generally a lawyer who offers free help with estate planning, the establishment of living wills, and the power of attorney.

The term *patient advocate* usually describes the person who receives the power of attorney on behalf of the patient. The patient advocate ensures that the patient's wishes regarding life-sustaining treatment, funeral arrangements, and so on, are carried out as instructed. The patient advocate is the patient's legally designated representative, taking precedence over even the family.

The Gay Men's Health Crisis has greatly centralized volunteer efforts in Manhattan; other volunteer approaches differ regionally. In San Francisco, for example, there is a greater tendency for a number of smaller organizations to each focus on one issue, working together to form a safety net for individuals in need.

Hotlines are always in need of well-informed and empathic individuals. Some hotlines focus on crisis intervention, while others serve as information sources. Religious support is often lacking, primarily because many infected people have been ostracized from traditional social channels, including religious networks. Selected patients would benefit from religious support. Hospitals also have traditionally relied on volunteers. In hospitals, volunteers perform varied tasks, allowing nurses to concentrate on nursing interventions.

The need for volunteers keeps growing and diversifying. The efforts of both skilled and unskilled workers are needed; anyone with heart will find a welcome place.

APPENDIX A:

Revision of the CDC Surveillance Case Definition for Acquired Immunodeficiency Syndrome.

For national reporting, a case of AIDS is defined as an illness characterized by one or more of the following "indicator" diseases, depending on the status of laboratory evidence of HIV infection, as shown below.

CDC Appendix I

I. **Without Laboratory Evidence Regarding HIV Infection**

    If laboratory tests for HIV were not performed or gave inconclusive results (*See* Appendix I) and the patient had no other cause of immunodeficiency listed in Section I.A below, then any disease listed in Section I.B indicates AIDS if it was diagnosed by a definitive method (*See* Appendix II).

    A. Causes of immunodeficiency that disqualify diseases as indicators of AIDS in the absence of laboratory evidence for HIV infection
        1. high-dose or long-term systemic corticosteroid therapy or other immunosuppressive/cytotoxic therapy ≥ 3 months before the onset of the indicator disease
        2. any of the following diseases diagnosed ≥ 3 months after diagnosis of the indicator disease: Hodgkin's disease, non-Hodgkin's lymphoma (other than primary brain lymphoma), lymphocytic leukemia, multiple myeloma, any other cancer of lymphoreticular or histiocytic tissue, or angioimmunoblastic lymphadenopathy
        3. a genetic (congenital) immunodeficiency syndrome or an acquired immunodeficiency syndrome atypical of HIV infection, such as one involving hypogammaglobulinemia

    B. Indicator diseases diagnosed definitively (*See* Appendix II)
        1. candidiasis of the esophagus, trachea, bronchi, or lungs
        2. cryptococcosis, extrapulmonary
        3. cryptosporidiosis with diarrhea persisting >1 month
        4. cytomegalovirus disease of an organ other than liver, spleen, or lymph nodes in a patient >1 month of age
        5. herpes simplex virus infection causing a mucocutaneous ulcer that persists longer than 1 month; or bronchitis, pneumonitis, or esophagitis for any duration affecting a patient >1 month of age
        6. Kaposi's sarcoma affecting a patient <60 years of age
        7. lymphoma of the brain (primary) affecting a patient <60 years of age
        8. lymphoid interstitial pneumonia and/or pulmonary lymphoid hyperplasia (LIP/PLH complex) affecting a child <13 years of age
        9. *Mycobacterium avium* complex or *M. kansasii* disease, disseminated (lat a site other than or in addition to lungs, skin, or cervical or hilar lymph nodes)
        10. *Pneumocystis carinii* pneumonia
        11. progressive multifocal leukoencephalopathy
        12. toxoplasmosis of the brain affecting a patient >1 month of age

II. **With Laboratory Evidence for HIV Infection** *Regardless of the presence of other causes of immunodeficiency (I.A),* in the presence of laboratory evidence for HIV infection (*See* Appendix I), any disease listed above (I.B) or below (II.A or II.B) indicates a diagnosis of AIDS.

    A. Indicator diseases diagnosed definitively (*See* Appendix II)
        1. bacterial infections, multiple or recurrent (any combination of at least two within a 2-year period), of the following types affecting a child <13 years of age: septicemia, pneumonia, meningitis, bone or joint infection, or abscess of an internal organ or body cavity (excluding otitis media or superficial skin or mucosal abscesses), caused by *Haemophilus, Streptococcus* (including pneumococcus), or other pyogenic bacteria

2. coccidioidomycosis, disseminated (at a site other than or in addition to lungs or cervical or hilar lymph nodes)
3. HIV encephalopathy (also called "HIV dementia," "AIDS dementia," or "subacute encephalitis due to HIV") (*See* Appendix II for description)
4. histoplasmosis, disseminated (at a site other than or in addition to lungs or cervical or hilar lymph nodes)
5. isosporiasis with diarrhea persisting >1 month
6. Kaposi's sarcoma at any age
7. lymphoma of the brain (primary) at any age
8. other non-Hodgkin's lymphoma of B-cell or unknown immunologic phenotype and the following histologic types:
   a. small noncleaved lymphoma (either Burkitt or non-Burkitt type) (*See* Appendix IV for equivalent terms and numeric codes used in the *International Classification of Diseases,* Ninth Revision, Clinical Modification)
   b. immunoblastic sarcoma (equivalent to any of the following, although not necessarily all in combination: immunoblastic lymphoma, large-cell lymphoma, diffuse histiocytic lymphoma, diffuse undifferentiated lymphoma, or high-grade lymphoma) (*See* Appendix IV for equivalent terms and numeric codes used in the *International Classification of Diseases,* Ninth Revision, Clinical Modification)
   Note: Lymphomas are not included here if they are of T-cell immunologic phenotype or their histologic type is not described or is described as "lymphocytic," "lymphoblastic," "small cleaved," or "plasmacytoid lymphocytic"
9. any mycobacterial disease caused by mycobacteria other than *M. tuberculosis,* disseminated (at a site other than or in addition to lungs, skin, or cervical or hilar lymph nodes)
10. disease caused by *M. tuberculosis,* extrapulmonary (involving at least one site outside the lungs, regardless of whether there is concurrent pulmonary involvement)
11. *Salmonella* (nontyphoid) septicemia, recurrent
12. HIV wasting syndrome (emaciation, "slim disease") (*See* Appendix II for description)

B. Indicator diseases diagnosed presumptively (by a method other than those in Appendix II)

   Note: Given the seriousness of diseases indicative of AIDS, it is generally important to diagnose them definitively, especially when therapy that would be used may have serious side effects or when definitive diagnosis is needed for eligibility for antiretroviral therapy. Nonetheless, in some situations, a patient's condition will not permit the performance of definitive tests. In other situations, accepted clinical practice may be to diagnose presumptively based on the presence of characteristic clinical and laboratory abnormalities. Guidelines for presumptive diagnoses are suggested in Appendix III.

   1. candidiasis of the esophagus
   2. cytomegalovirus retinitis with loss of vision
   3. Kaposi's sarcoma
   4. lymphoid interstitial pneumonia and/or pulmonary lymphoid hyperplasia (LIP/PLH complex) affecting a child <13 years of age
   5. mycobacterial disease (acid-fast bacilli with species not identified by culture), disseminated (involving at least one site other than or in addition to lungs, skin, or cervical or hilar lymph nodes)
   6. *Pneumocystis carinii* pneumonia
   7. toxoplasmosis of the brain affecting a patient >1 month of age

III. **With Laboratory Evidence Against HIV Infection**
With laboratory test results negative for HIV infection (*See* Appendix I), a diagnosis of AIDS for surveillance purposes is ruled out *unless:*

A. all the other causes of immunodeficiency listed above in Section I.A are excluded;
   AND
B. the patient has had either:
   1. *Pneumocystis carinii* pneumonia diagnosed by a definitive method (*See* Appendix II); **OR**
   2.
   a. any of the other diseases indicative of AIDS listed above in Section I.B diagnosed by

a definitive method (*See* Appendix II); **AND**
    b.   a T-helper/inducer (CD4) lymphocyte count <400/mm₃.

CDC Appendix II

Definitive Diagnostic Methods for Diseases Indicative of AIDS

Diseases	Definitive Diagnostic Methods

cryptosporidiosis
cytomegalovirus
isosporiasis
Kaposi's sarcoma
lymphoma
lymphoid pneumonia or
  hyperplasia
Pneumocystis carinii
  pneumonia
progressive multifocal
  leukoencephalopathy
toxoplasmosis
	microscopy (histology or cytology)

candidiasis.	gross inspection by endoscopy or autopsy or by microscopy (histology or cytology) on a specimen obtained directly from the tissues affected (including scrapings from the mucosal surface), not from a culture.
coccidioidomycosis	microscopy (histology or cytology), culture, or detection of antigen in a specimen obtained directly from the tissues affected or a fluid from those tissues.
cryptococcosis herpes simplex virus histoplasmosis	
tuberculosis other mycobacteriosis salmonellosis. other bacterial infection	culture.
HIV encephalopathy* (dementia)	clinical findings of disabling cognitive and/or motor dysfunction interfering with occupation or activities of daily living, or loss of behavioral developmental milestones affecting a child, progressing over weeks to months, in the absence of a concurrent illness or condition other than HIV infection that could explain the findings. Methods to rule out such concurrent illnesses and conditions must include cerebrospinal fluid examination and either brain imaging (computed tomography or magnetic resonance) or autopsy.
HIV wasting syndrome*	findings of profound involuntary weight loss >10% of baseline body weight plus either chronic diarrhea (at least two loose stools per day for ≥ 30 days) or chronic weakness and documented fever (for ≥ 30 days, intermittent or constant) in the absence of a concurrent illness or condition other than HIV infection that could explain the findings (e.g., cancer, tuberculosis, cryptosporidiosis, or other specific enteritis).

*For HIV encephalopathy and HIV wasting syndrome, the methods of diagnosis described here are not truly definitive, but are sufficiently rigorous for surveillance purposes.

FIGURE I. Flow diagram for revised CDC case definition of AIDS, September 1, 1987

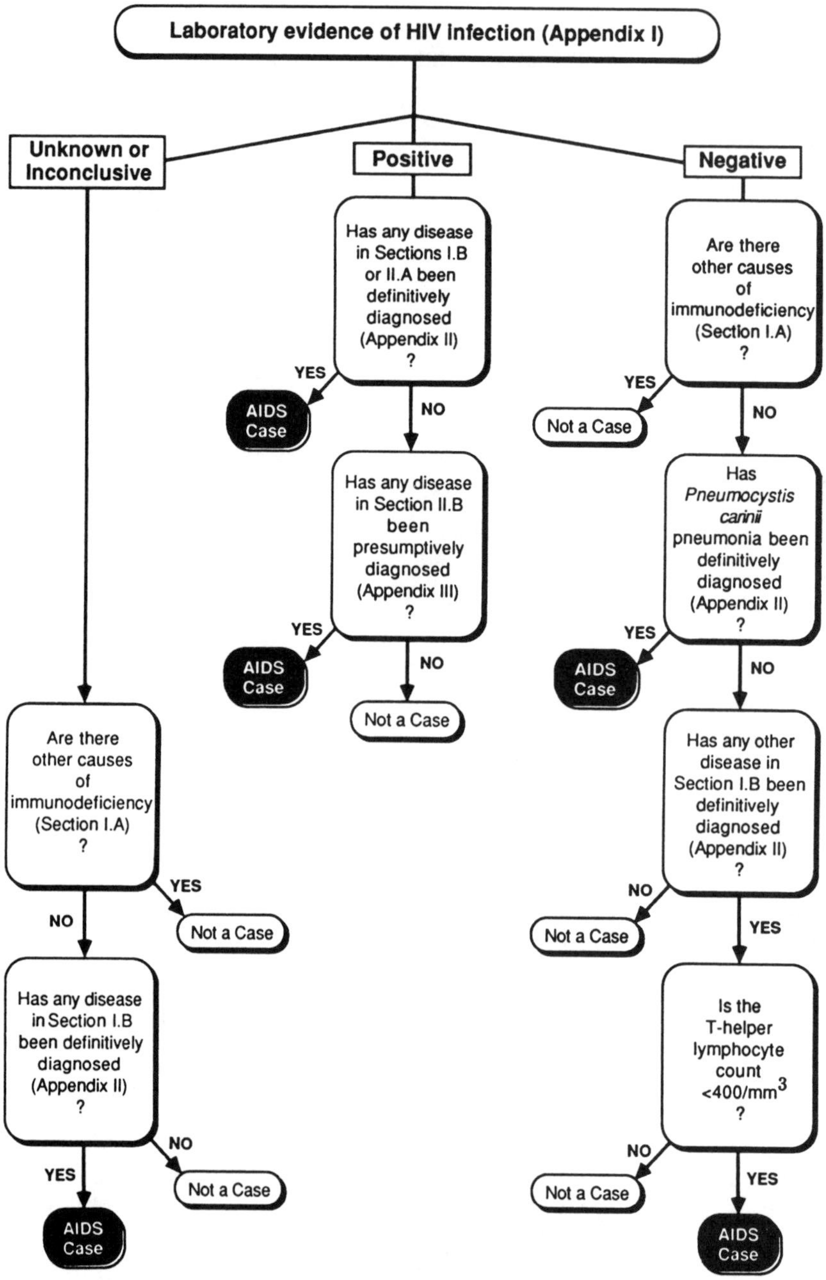

CDC Appendix III

Suggested Guidelines for Presumptive Diagnosis
of Diseases Indicative of AIDS

Diseases	Presumptive Diagnositic Criteria
candidiasis of esophagus.	a. recent onset of retrosternal pain on swallowing; **AND** b. oral candidiasis diagnosed by the gross appearance of white patches or plaques on an erythematous base or by the microscopic appearance of fungal mycelial filaments in an uncultured specimen scraped from the oral mucosa.
cytomegalovirus retinitis.	a characteristic appearance on serial ophthalmoscopic examinations (e.g., discrete patches of retinal whitening with distinct borders, spreading in a centrifugal manner, following blood vessels, progressing over several months, frequently associated with retinal vasculitis, hemorrhage, and necrosis). Resolution of active disease leaves retinal scarring and atrophy with retinal pigment epithelial mottling.
mycobacteriosis.	microscopy of a specimen from stool or normally sterile body fluids or tissue from a site other than lungs, skin, or cervical or hilar lymph nodes, showing acid-fast bacilli of a species not identified by culture.
Kaposi's sarcoma.	a characteristic gross appearance of an erythematous or violaceous plaque-like lesion on skin or mucous membrane. **Note:** Presumptive diagnosis of Kaposi's sarcoma should not be made by clinicians who have seen few cases of it.
lymphoid interstitial pneumonia.	bilateral reticulonodular interstitial pulmonary infiltrates present on chest X-ray for ≥ 2 months with no pathogen identified and no response to antibiotic treatment.
Pneumocystis carinii pneumonia.	a. a history of dyspnea on exertion or nonproductive cough of recent onset (within the past 3 months); **AND** b. chest X-ray evidence of diffuse bilateral interstitial infiltrates or gallium scan evidence of diffuse bilateral pulmonary disease; AND c. arterial blood gas analysis showing an arterial pO_2 of <70 mm Hg or a low respiratory diffusing capacity (<80% of predicted values) or an increase in the alveolar-arterial oxygen tension gradient; **AND** d. no evidence of a bacterial pneumonia.
toxoplasmosis of the brain.	a. recent onset of a focal neurologic abnormality consistent with intracranial disease or a reduced level of consciousness; **AND** b. brain imaging evidence of a lesion having a mass effect (on computed tomography or nuclear magnetic resonance) or the radiographic appearance of which is enhanced by injection of contrast medium; **AND** c. serum antibody to toxoplasmosis or successful response to therapy for toxoplasmosis.

Adapted from

MMWR 1987 August; 36:4S-6S, 11S-14S

Centers for Disease Control

Atlanta, Georgia 30333

APPENDIX B:

Education and Foster Care of Children Infected with Human T-Lymphotropic Virus Type III/Lymphadenopathy-Associated Virus.

Risk of Transmission in the School, Day-Care or Foster-Care Setting

None of the identified cases of HTLV-III/LAV infection in the United States are known to have been transmitted in the school, day-care, or foster-care setting or through other casual person-to-person contact. Other than the sexual partners of HTLV-III/LAV-infected patients and infants born to infected mothers, none of the family members of the over 12,000 AIDS patients reported to CDC have been reported to have AIDS. Six studies of family members of patients with HTLV-III/LAV infection have failed to demonstrate HTLV-III/LAV transmission to adults who were not sexual contacts of the infected patients or to older children who were not likely at risk from perinatal transmission (6–11).

Based on current evidence, casual person-to-person contact as would occur among school-children appears to pose no risk. However, studies of the risk of transmission through contact between younger children and neurologically handicapped children who lack control of their body secretions are very limited. Based on experience with other communicable diseases, a theoretical potential for transmission would be greatest among these children. It should be emphasized that any theoretical transmission would most likely involve exposure of open skin lesions or mucous membranes to blood and possibly other body fluids of an infected person.

Risks to the Child with HTLV-III/LAV Infection

HTLV-III/LAV infection may result in immunodeficiency. Such children may have a greater risk of encountering infectious agents in a school or day-care setting than at home. Foster homes with multiple children may also increase the risk. In addition, younger children and neurologically handicapped children who may display behaviors such as mouthing of toys would be expected to be at greater risk for acquiring infections. Immunodepressed children are also at greater risk of suffering severe complications from such infections as chickenpox, cytomegalovirus, tuberculosis, herpes simplex, and measles. Assessment of the risk to the immunodepressed child is best made by the child's physician who is aware of the child's immune status. The risk of acquiring some infections, such as chickenpox, may be reduced by prompt use of specific immune globulin following a known exposure.

RECOMMENDATIONS

1. Decisions regarding the type of educational and care setting for HTLV-III/LAV-infected children should be based on the behavior, neurologic development, and physical condition of the child and the expected type of interaction with others in that setting. These decisions are best made using the team approach including the child's physician, public health personnel, the child's parent or guardian, and personnel associated with the proposed care or educational setting. In each case, risks and benefits to both the infected child and to others in the setting should be weighed.
2. For most infected school-aged children, the benefits of an unrestricted setting would outweigh the risks of their acquiring potentially harmful infections in the setting and the apparent nonexistent risk of transmission of HTLV-III/LAV. These children should be allowed to attend school and after-school day-care and to be placed in a foster home in an unrestricted setting.
3. For the infected preschool-aged child and for some neurologically handicapped children who lack control of their body secretions or who display behavior, such as biting, and those children who have uncoverable, oozing lesions, a more restricted environment is advisable until more is known about transmission in these settings. Children infected with HTLV-III/LAV should be cared for and educated in settings that minimize exposure of other children to blood or body fluids.
4. Care involving exposure to the infected child's body fluids and excrement, such as feeding and diaper changing, should be performed by persons who are aware of the child's HTLV-III/LAV infection and the modes of possible transmission. In any setting involving an HTLV-

III/LAV-infected person, good handwashing after exposure to blood and body fluids and before caring for another child should be observed, and gloves should be worn if open lesions are present on the caretaker's hands. Any open lesions on the infected person should also be covered.

5. Because other infections in addition to HTLV-III/LAV can be present in blood or body fluids, all schools and day-care facilities, regardless of whether children with HTLV-III/LAV infection are attending, should adopt routine procedures for handling blood or body fluids. Soiled surfaces should be promptly cleaned with disinfectants, such as household bleach (diluted 1 part bleach to 10 parts water). Disposable towels or tissues should be used whenever possible, and mops should be rinsed in the disinfectant. Those who are cleaning should avoid exposure of open skin lesions or mucous membranes to the blood or body fluids.

6. The hygienic practices of children with HTLV-III/LAV infection may improve as the child matures. Alternatively, the hygienic practices may deteriorate if the child's condition worsens. Evaluation to assess the need for a restricted environment should be performed regularly.

7. Physicians caring for children born to mothers with AIDS or at increased risk of acquiring HTLV-III/LAV infection should consider testing the children for evidence of HTLV-III/LAV infection for medical reasons. For example, vaccination of infected children with live virus vaccines, such as the measles-mumps-rubella vaccine (MMR), may be hazardous. These children also need to be followed closely for problems with growth and development and given prompt and aggressive therapy for infections and exposure to potentially lethal infections, such as varicella. In the event that an antiviral agent or other therapy for HTLV-III/LAV infection becomes available, these children should be considered for such therapy. Knowledge that a child is infected will allow parents and other caretakers to take precautions when exposed to the blood and body fluids of the child.

8. Adoption and foster-care agencies should consider adding HTLV-III/LAV screening to their routine medical evaluations of children at increased risk of infection before placement in the foster or adoptive home, since these parents must make decisions regarding the medical care of the child and must consider the possible social and psychological effects on their families.

9. Mandatory screening as a condition for school entry is not warranted based on available data.

10. Persons involved in the care and education of HTLV-III/LAV-infected children should respect the child's right to privacy, including maintaining confidential records. The number of personnel who are aware of the child's condition should be kept at a minimum needed to assure proper care of the child and to detect situations where the potential for transmission may increase (e.g., bleeding injury).

11. All educational and public health departments, regardless of whether HTLV-III/LAV-infected children are involved, are strongly encouraged to inform parents, children, and educators regarding HTLV-III/LAV and its transmission. Such education would greatly assist efforts to provide the best care and education for infected children while minimizing the risk of transmission to others.

Adapted from
MMWR 1985 August 30;34: 517-521
Centers for Disease Control
Atlanta, Georgia 30333

APPENDIX C:

Recommendations for Prevention of HIV Transmission in Health-Care Settings

Precautions to Prevent Transmission of HIV

Universal Precautions

Since medical history and examination cannot reliably identify all patients infected with HIV or other blood-borne pathogens, blood and body-fluid precautions should be consistently used for **all** patients. This approach, previously recommended by CDC (3,4), and referred to as "universal blood and body-fluid precautions" or "universal precautions," should be used in the care of **all** patients, especially including those in emergency-care settings in which the risk of blood exposure is increased and the infection status of the patient is usually unknown (20).

1. All health-care workers should routinely use appropriate barrierprecautions to prevent skin and mucous-membrane exposure when contact withblood or other body fluids of any patient is anticipated. Gloves should be worn for touching blood and body fluids, mucous membranes, or non-intact skin of all patients, for handling items or surfaces soiled with blood or body fluids, and for performing venipuncture and other vascular access procedures. Gloves should be changed after contact with each patient. Masks and protective eyewear or face shields should be worn during procedures that are likely to generate droplets of blood or other body fluids to prevent exposure of mucous membranes of the mouth, nose, and eyes. Gowns or aprons should be worn during procedures that are likely to generate splashes of blood or other body fluids.

2. Hands and other skin surfaces should be washed immediately and thoroughly if contaminated with blood or other body fluids. Hands should be washed immediately after gloves are removed.

3. All health-care workers should take precautions to prevent injuries caused by needles, scalpels, and other sharp instruments or devices during procedures; when cleaning used instruments; during disposal of used needles; and when handling sharp instruments after procedures. To prevent needlestick injuries, needles should not be recapped, purposely bent or broken by hand, removed from disposable syringes, or otherwise manipulated by hand. After they are used, disposable syringes and needles, scalpel blades, and other sharp items should be placed in puncture-resistant containers for disposal; the puncture-resistant containers should be located as close as practical to the use area. Large-bore reusable needles should be placed in a puncture-resistant container for transport to the reprocessing area.

4. Although saliva has not been implicated in HIV trasmission, to minimize the need for emergency mouth-to-mouth resuscitation, mouthpieces, resuscitation bags, or other ventilation devices should be available for use in areas in which the need for resuscitation is predictable.

5. Health-care workers who have exudative lesions or weeping dermatitis should refrain from all direct patient care and from handling patient-care equipment until the condition resolves.

6. Pregnant health-care workers are not known to be at greater risk of contracting HIV infection than health-care workers who are not pregnant; however, if a health-care worker develops HIV infection during pregnancy, the infant is at risk of infection resulting from perinatal transmission. Because of this risk, pregnant health-care workers should be especially familiar with and strictly adhere to precautions to minimize the risk of HIV transmission.

Implementation of universal blood and body-fluid precautions for **all** patients eliminates the need for use of the isolation category of "Blood and Body Fluid Precautions" previously recommended by CDC (7) for patients known or suspected to be infected with blood-borne pathogens. Isolation precautions (e.g., enteric, "AFB" [7]) should be used as necessary if associated conditions, such as infectious diarrhea or tuberculosis, are diagnosed or suspected.

Precautions for Dentistry

Blood, saliva, and gingival fluid from **all** dental patients should be considered infective. Special emphasis should be placed on the following precautions for preventing transmission of blood-borne pathogens in dental practice in both institutional and non-institutional settings.

1. In addition to wearing gloves for contact with oral mucous membranes of all patients, all dental workers should wear surgical masks and protective eyewear or chin-length plastic face shields during dental procedures in which splashing or spattering of blood, saliva, or gingival fluids is likely. Rubber dams, high-speed evacuation, and proper patient positioning, when appropriate, should be utilized to minimize generation of droplets and spatter.

2. Handpieces should be sterilized after use with each patient, since blood, saliva, or gingival fluid of patients may be aspirated into the handpiece or waterline. Handpieces that cannot be sterilized should at least be flushed, the outside surface cleaned and wiped with a suitable chemical germicide, and then rinsed. Handpieces should be flushed at the beginning of the day and after use with each patient. Manufacturers' recommendations should be followed for use and maintenance of waterlines and check valves and for flushing of handpieces. The same precautions should be used for ultrasonic scalers and air/water syringes.

3. Blood and saliva should be thoroughly and carefully cleaned from material that has been used in the mouth (e.g., impression materials, bite registration), especially before polishing and grinding intra-oral devices. Contaminated materials, impressions, and intra-oral devices should also be cleaned and disinfected before being handled in the dental laboratory and before they are placed in the patient's mouth. Because of the increasing variety of dental materials used intra-orally, dental workers should consult with manufacturers as to the stability of specific materials when using disinfection procedures.

4. Dental equipment and surfaces that are difficult to disinfect (e.g., light handles or X-ray-unit heads) and that may become contaminated should be wrapped with impervious-backed paper, aluminum foil, or clear plastic wrap. The coverings should be removed and discarded, and clean coverings should be put in place after use with each patient.

Precautions for Autopsies or Morticians' Services

In addition to the universal blood and body-fluid precautions listed above, the following precautions should be used by persons performing postmortem procedures:

1. All persons performing or assisting in postmortem procedures should wear gloves, masks, protective eyewear, gowns, and waterproof aprons.

2. Instruments and surfaces contaminated during postmortem procedures should be decontaminated with an appropriate chemical germicide.

Precautions for Dialysis

Patients with end-stage renal disease who are undergoing maintenance dialysis and who have HIV infection can be dialyzed in hospital-based or free-standing dialysis units using conventional infection-control precautions (27). Universal blood and body-fluid precautions should be used when dialyzing **all** patients.

Strategies for disinfecting the dialysis fluid pathways of the hemodialysis machine are targeted to control bacterial contamination and generally consist of using 500–750 parts per million (ppm) of sodium hypochlorite (household bleach) for 30–40 minutes or 1.5%–2.0% formaldehyde overnight. In addition, several chemical germicides formulated to disinfect dialysis machines are commercially available. None of these protocols or procedures need to be changed for dialyzing patients infected with HIV.

Patients infected with HIV can be dialyzed by either hemodialysis or peritoneal dialysis and do not need to be isolated from other patients. The type of dialysis treatment (i.e., hemodialysis or peritoneal dialysis) should be based on the needs of the patient. The dialyzer may be discarded after each use. Alternatively, centers that reuse dialyzers—i.e., a specific single-use dialyzer is issued to a specific patient, removed, cleaned, disinfected, and reused several times on the same patient only—may include HIV-infected patients in the dialyzer-reuse program. An individual dialyzer must never be used on more than one patient.

Precautions for Laboratories

Blood and other body fluids from **all** patients should be considered infective. To supplement the universal blood and body-fluid precautions listed above, the following precautions are recommended for health-care workers in clinical laboratories.

1. All specimens of blood and body fluids should be put in a well-constructed container with a secure lid to prevent leaking during transport. Care should be taken when collecting each specimen to avoid contaminating the outside of the container and of the laboratory form accompanying the specimen.

2. All persons processing blood and body-fluid specimens (e.g., removing tops from vacuum tubes) should wear gloves. Masks and protective eyewear should be worn if mucous-membrane contact with blood or body fluids is anticipated. Gloves should be changed and hands washed after completion of specimen processing.

3. For routine procedures, such as histologic and pathologic studies or microbiologic culturing, a biological safety cabinet is not necessary. However, biological safety cabinets (Class I or II) should be used whenever procedures are conducted that have a high potential for generating droplets. These include activities such as blending, sonicating, and vigorous mixing.

4. Mechanical pipetting devices should be used for manipulating all liquids in the laboratory. Mouth pipetting must not be done.

5. Use of needles and syringes should be limited to situations in which there is no alternative, and the recommendations for preventing injuries with needles outlined under universal precautions should be followed.

6. Laboratory work surfaces should be decontaminated with an appropriate chemical germicide after a spill of blood or other body fluids and when work activities are completed.

7. Contaminated materials used in laboratory tests should be decontaminated before reprocessing or be placed in bags and disposed of in accordance with institutional policies for disposal of infective waste (24).

8. Scientific equipment that has been contaminated with blood or other body fluids should be decontaminated and cleaned before being repaired in the laboratory or transported to the manufacturer.

9. All persons should wash their hands after completing laboratory activities and should remove protective clothing before leaving the laboratory.

Implementation of universal blood and body-fluid precautions for **all** patients eliminates the need for warning labels on specimens since blood and other body fluids from all patients should be considered infective.

Management of Infected Health-Care Workers

Health-care workers with impaired immune systems resulting from HIV infection or other causes are at increased risk of acquiring or experiencing serious complications of infectious disease. Of particular concern is the risk of severe infection following exposure to patients with infectious diseases that are easily transmitted if appropriate precautions are not taken (e.g., measles, varicella). Any health-care worker with an impaired immune system should be counseled about the potential risk associated with taking care of patients with any transmissible infection and should continue to follow existing recommendations for infection control to minimize risk of exposure to other infectious agents (7,35). Recommendations of the Immunization Practices Advisory Committee (ACIP) and institutional policies concerning requirements for vaccinating health-care workers with live-virus vaccines (e.g., measles, rubella) should also be considered.

The question of whether workers infected with HIV—especially those who perform invasive procedures—can adequately and safely be allowed to perform patient-care duties or whether their work assignments should be changed must be determined on an individual basis. These decisions should be made by the health-care worker's personal physician(s) in conjunction with the medical directors and personnel health service staff of the employing institution or hospital.

Management of Exposures

If a health-care worker has a parenteral (e.g., needlestick or cut) or mucous-membrane (e.g., splash to the eye or mouth) exposure to blood or other body fluids or has a cutaneous exposure involving large amounts of blood or prolonged contact with blood—especially when the exposed skin is chapped, abraded, or afflicted with dermatitis—the source patient should be informed of the incident and tested for serologic evidence of HIV infection after consent is obtained. Policies should be developed for testing source patients in situations in which consent cannot be obtained (e.g., an unconscious patient).

If the source patient has AIDS, is positive for HIV antibody, or refuses the test, the health-care workers should be counseled regarding the risk of infection and evaluated clinically and serologically for evidence of HIV infection as soon as possible after the exposure. The health-care worker should be advised to report and seek medical evaluation for any acute febrile illness that occurs within 12 weeks after the exposure. Such an illness—particularly one characterized by fever, rash, or lymphadenopathy—may be indicative of recent HIV infection. Seronegative health-care workers should be retested 6 weeks post-exposure and on a periodic basis thereafter (e.g., 12 weeks and 6 months after exposure) to determine whether transmission has occurred. During this follow-up period—especially the first 6–12 weeks after exposure, when most infected persons are expected to seroconvert—exposed health-care workers should follow U.S. Public Health Service (PHS) recommendations for preventing transmission of HIV (36,37).

No further follow-up of a health-care worker exposed to infection as described above is necessary if the source patient is seronegative unless the source patient is at high risk of HIV infection. In the latter case, a subsequent specimen (e.g., 12 weeks following exposure) may be obtained from the health-care worker for antibody testing. If the source patient cannot be identified, decisions regarding appropriate follow-up should be individualized. Serologic testing should be available to all health-care workers who are concerned that they may have been infected with HIV.

If a patient has a parenteral or mucous-membrane exposure to blood or other body fluid of a health-care worker, the patient should be informed of the incident, and the same procedure outlined above for management of exposures should be followed for both the source health-care worker and the exposed patient.

Adapted from
MMWR 1987 August 21: 36/2S
Centers for Disease Control
Atlanta, Georgia 30333

INDEX